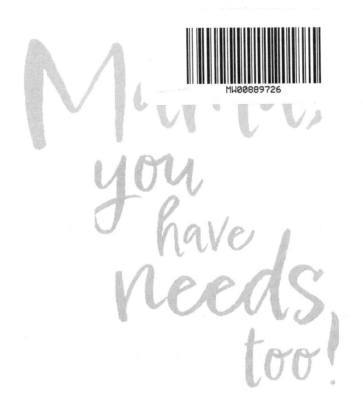

Mama, you have needs, too!

Self-Care, Fitness, and Nutrition for New Moms

Stephanie Baier

ISBN: 9798799698492
Published by Project Create LLC 2021

Contents

Special Bonus!

Want the companion journal for free?

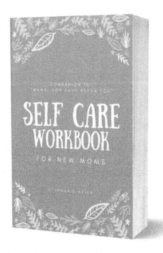

Get FREE, unlimited access to this and more books and resources by joining our community!

SCAN WITH YOUR CAMERA TO GET YOUR WORKBOOK!

Introduction

You've just left the hospital with your beautiful new baby in your arms, and you couldn't be more content. Everyone says the first few weeks are rough, but you know it will be worth it. What could possibly go wrong?

Fast forward several months. You're hardly sleeping, you're an emotional wreck, and you're going to lose it if you can't get some time to yourself. Perhaps, you've been trying and trying to lose the weight you gained during your pregnancy. You go for long walks with your baby every day and you are diligently counting calories, but the numbers on the scale aren't budging. To top things off, you are constantly hungry, and your baby wants to be held all the time. It feels almost impossible to feed yourself a decent meal, let alone a healthy one.

Your mom, well-meaning strangers, and your OB-GYN constantly tell you to get more sleep, make sure you're eating well-balanced meals, and drink lots of water. But every time someone offers you a bit of advice, you want to throw your hands to the sky and shout, "BUT HOW???" Where is the time? Where is the energy? And why in the world are my current efforts doing nothing?

You love your baby, and taking the time to care for your health will do both of you a favor. You will be able to provide important nutrition to your infant (if you are breastfeeding), and you will have the mental and physical resources to really be there for your little one.

This 30-day guide has been simplified so you can easily implement it into your daily routine with baby. I'm here to help you feel more calm, collected, and confident in your health! I am a young mom, so believe me, I know how you're feeling, and I can tell you that it *is* possible to feel great again!

I also want to preface this book by stating that your body likely won't ever return to its pre-pregnancy state. Bearing a child is a huge ordeal! But this certainly does not mean that your body will never be healthy and strong again. It can, and it will! And your mental health will improve right along with it. Mental and physical health are, after all, tightly connected.

If you are trying to get back to your pre-pregnancy weight, it's important to understand that the reason your body is holding on to excess fat is unique, and therefore requires a unique solution. Think of it this way. Imagine that a certain mechanic (we will call him Dave) loses some functionality in his car. He tries a few fixes without any improvement until finally he replaces the drive belt, and the car is once more running smoothly. Dave decides that replacing the drive belt must be the way to cure all car troubles and applies the same treatment to every car that enters his shop for repairs. While it's obvious what's wrong with this idea, we frequently apply the same logic to weight loss. We erroneously assume that if it works for Jane, it will work for everyone else. We forget that our bodies are unique, and we all experience kinks in our health for different reasons. Dave cannot assume that a faulty drive belt is the problem with every car he fixes any more than we can assume that the same treatment will make everyone lose weight. So, if you find your body is holding on to excess weight, we need to determine what is broken. What is preventing your body from running smoothly and assuming its optimal health? Is it stress? Is it a time restriction? Is it related to body image, activity levels, motivation, or diet? Family culture? Home or work environment?

Of course, if you suffer from a medical condition such as diabetes, hypothyroidism, or PCOS, you should work closely with a medical professional to determine the best route to weight loss. Some physiological conditions make weight loss difficult, but not impossible.

Over the next 30 days, you will learn the basic science behind diet, health, and weight loss and why some strategies work more than others. You will adjust your mindset to find peace where you are at right now and re-discover positivity and enthusiasm in your daily progression. You will evaluate your priorities, set goals, and implement small, gradual, and permanent lifestyle changes. You can, and you will, live a healthier life!

Read each section in the morning, or the night before if needed. Each chapter will include a positive affirmation to repeat to yourself throughout the day. You will then learn a little about diet and health and receive a daily challenge. This will be your focus for the next 24 hours. Our goal is to simplify the steps you can take to a healthier lifestyle.

You only need to focus on and apply one thing at a time. I would highly recommend keeping a journal and recording your thoughts at the end of each day. (See page 1 for access to a free companion workbook/journal!) Write down what went well, what you learned, and what you would like to continue or repeat. At the end of the 30 days, I hope you will have a better idea of what permanent lifestyle changes you would like to make and better understand what impact they have on your health. Pay attention to the actions and challenges that seem to impact your health the most. Try to pinpoint what is broken, that thing that is holding you back from your optimal health.

And above all, know that you are not alone in your journey! We all struggle with the first year to some degree, though each experience is a little different. Remember that the healthy habits you develop over the next 30 days should lead to *permanent* lifestyle changes that are 100%

worth your while. Caring for your health will benefit not only you but also the health of your babies. Your kids will follow the healthy habits you develop now, and as stated previously, you will have the resources to be the best mom you can be.

It won't be perfect. Each day brings its blessings and its challenges. Your health and your life look different now that you have a little one by your side. You will need to make adjustments based around the needs of your baby. This may mean that you have a week here and there where you don't exercise, or you reach out for help with meals. The following tips are here to guide you and educate you. I don't want you to stress when things don't go perfectly!

Recipe Cards Key

Each recipe includes a recipe card. At the bottom right corner of each card, you will find five color-coded numbers representing the following macronutrients:

Protein (first number on the right)

Fat (second number)

Carbohydrates (third number)

Fiber (fourth number)

Sugar (fifth number)

The First Weeks Postpartum

You've just left the hospital, holding a beautiful, brand-new baby. You can't help but smile as you gaze down at your precious little package. But now that you're leaving the care of the hospital staff, or your midwife, you realize you have no idea what's next! Not to mention the fact that labor is over, but you are still in pain. Why did no one mention the discomforts that follow delivery?

The first week after giving birth is both magical and difficult, but nothing you can't handle! Each week that follows brings new challenges and blessings. Your experience won't be exactly like everyone else's, but rest assured, you are not alone in your journey. Here are a few things to be aware of ahead of time (and some resources to handle them) so you can forget the discomforts and enjoy every moment cuddling your sweet baby!

If you are still preparing for childbirth, check out the resources at the end of this chapter. I compiled a list of things I did and learned preparatory to having an unmedicated birth, including diet, exercises, stretches, meditation, and more. I also included a link to my first birth experience!

I Just Went Through the Pains of Labor. Why Do I Still Hurt?

Giving birth is a major event. And your body will need some time to recover! It surprised me to find out that the bleeding could take up to six weeks to stop. For me it took five, which is much longer than a period!

Some things to look forward to:

The "shakes." Giving birth is such an ordeal, that your body almost seems to go into shock once the baby is out. But it is perfectly normal to be rather shaky following birth. Stay warm and rest up, and the shakes will go away soon.

Tearing: I didn't tear with my first birth, but I had some minor abrasions, little tears that didn't need stitches. And they still stung! At the hospital or birth center, you will be given a squirt bottle to squirt gently on yourself when you need to pee. This dilutes the urine, so it stings less on your cuts.

Sitting is SO uncomfortable. Due to tearing, abrasions, or bruising, sitting will be nearly impossible for the first week or so. Go for soft pillows, avoid hard chairs, and rest lying down as much as possible to take pressure off the perineum (and to assist healing!). Apply a cold compress for the first 24hrs (or padsicles: pads filled with water and frozen) and take sitz baths in the days following: sit in a tub of warm water with dissolved Epsom salts. When I took sitz baths, I had to kneel in the water to reduce the pressure on my perineum. It wasn't the most comfortable position, but the warm water was soothing. You may also apply warm heat packs or rice packs and witch hazel to the swollen area.

Breastfeeding hurts at first. It's not as easy as it looks. For the first week, my nipples were insanely raw and sore. They bled and scabbed up, and I wanted to cry every time my baby girl needed to eat. And it doesn't help that infants spend a lot more time feeding when they're first born, because their stomachs are so tiny (so they need more frequent meals), and they're less efficient at taking out milk. So, my nipples hardly had time to rest from one feeding session to the next. Try applying some nipple cream to protect raw nipples, and *don't worry*! It will get better soon! If it doesn't, you can always see a lactation consultant to make sure your baby is getting a good latch. Gently pushing down on her chin as she eats, and giving her a breast "sandwich," are ways to make sure her lips flare open around the areola and most of the areola is in her mouth (not just the nipple). It hurts worse when her bottom lip is curled in as she sucks.

Breastfeeding triggers uterine contractions. Thought you were done with contractions? Turns out breastfeeding causes the uterus to contact down to its original size. This is *important*, but still uncomfortable. While the cramps are not as strong as they were in labor, they feel a lot like menstrual cramps. Your doctor may recommend taking ibuprofen or acetaminophen.

Your first few bowl movements are likely to be painful. There's something about pushing out a baby that makes your insides rather tender. It took me a few weeks to stop cringing when I needed to use the restroom. Use a stool softener like Colace (generic is fine), NOT a laxative, so you don't have to strain so much. Pushing is not super comfortable after birth! Make sure to get foods high in fiber and drink lots of water. You can also try drinking 1/2 cup apple juice with 1/2 cup prune juice, *warm.*

Hot, cold, and sweaty. For the first few days after giving birth, my body could not seem to regulate its temperature at all. When I was holding my baby, I was hot and sweaty, but as soon as someone else took her, I was absolutely freezing. I would shake like crazy until I'd snuggled under a massive pile of blankets for several minutes. And whether I was hot or cold, I was always ridiculously sweaty. I'm sure changing hormones and the process of recovery were to blame for this inconsistency.

Hungry and thirsty. Recovery burns energy, and if you are breastfeeding, you'll be sharing additional calories with your little one. For me, and for several friends I've talked with, the moment my baby starts eating, I get crazy hungry and thirsty. So, make sure to *keep a full water bottle and some snacks next to your bed* for feedings!

Hemorrhoids and infections. Giving birth can make your body more susceptible to infections such as UTIs, bladder infections, and yeast infections. Your doctor may prescribe you an antibiotic (for UTIs and bladder infections), and a special cream or oral antifungal drug for yeast infections. Hemorrhoids usually pop up from straining during a bowel movement (not to mention how much you strained during labor!). Witch Hazel hemorrhoidal wipes (found in many grocery stores) can be applied topically to reduce soreness. Also make sure to drink lots of water to reduce bladder/urinary tract infections. I started taking a women's probiotic and didn't have any more trouble with UTIs! Re-populating your body with healthy bacteria can help prevent bad bacteria from giving you trouble.

My Baby Does Not Want to Be Set Down!

Before I was sent home from the birth center, I was instructed to do five things: sleep, pee often, eat, nurse, and drink lots of water ("SPEND" acronym). What I didn't realize was how difficult it would be to complete such simple tasks with an infant! As soon as I set her down after a feeding, even if she was sound asleep, she'd wake up and fuss. I had to hold her to keep her content (not to mention that I sometimes had a hard time letting her go myself!). So, getting myself food was hard, refilling my water bottle was a chore, getting up to use the restroom was daunting, and sleeping was near impossible.

Luckily, I had lots of family support those first few weeks, so I didn't have to do it completely on my own. But slowly I found ways to do things one-handed, and my mom helped me acclimate baby to sleeping on her own so I could get some rest. Here are a few things to try:

First off, **just soak in each moment!** Your little one won't be so little forever, so enjoy holding her, snuggling, talking to her, taking lots of cute pictures, etc. It's okay if the dishes don't get done today. What's more important is that you are loving and bonding with your beautiful newborn!

Get a bassinet that can sit next to your bed or in your bed. This will be super helpful when you are exhausted at night and can hardly get up to retrieve your baby for nursing. It's also more comforting for baby to sleep near you!

Try a different sleeping position. Babies don't like to sleep on their backs. They love to be on their stomachs or their sides. They also love sleeping in swings, car seats, etc. because of the curved seat and head elevation. You'll need to keep an eye on them if they're in a swing or car seat, but this can be helpful if you need to set them down during the day. The safest position for a baby to sleep in is on his/her back, so please be very careful with this one. Consult your doctor, nurse, or OBGYN before making any adjustments to your little one's sleeping arrangements. Just be aware that if your baby doesn't seem to like sleeping on her back, she's completely normal! As soon as my baby was able to roll over onto her belly on her own, that was the only way she would sleep.

Comfort, then set baby back down for sleep. During the day when you have a bit more energy, try laying your infant down for a nap after a feeding. When she fusses, pick her up, hold, her, rock her, and set her back down again when she is asleep. If she wakes up again five minutes later, hold her again. This may not get your baby to sleep on her own right away, but slowly she may grow more comfortable with her own bed. We tried this and after about a month, she was sleeping longer stretches on her own (even up to five or six hours at night!).

Swaddle. Swaddling your baby can limit the *startle* reflex when she is lying down (which reflex can wake her up after she's fallen asleep). It also helps her feel more snug and secure, like she's back in the womb!

I've Fed Her and Am Trying to Soothe Her, but My Baby Is Still Crying. What Else Can I Do?

It can be frustrating when you've tried everything you know, and your baby is still unhappy. Here are a few final postpartum tips to help your little one adjust to life outside the womb.

Developmental spurts. Your child will go through periodic growth spurts. During this time, she will likely be fussier while eating (esp. if breast feeding, she will want milk faster than it is coming out now!). She will want to eat more frequently (cluster feeding, which will also increase your milk supply as she grows) and probably sleep for shorter intervals at night. She may just be fussier in general as her senses develop and new, unfamiliar sensations surround her.

Baby language. Did you know your baby has a language of her own? She may make specific noises based on her needs. For example, when she is hungry, she may cry out with a "neh" sound. This noise is caused by the sucking reflex.

Don't try to sleep train a newborn or let her "cry it out." Infants cannot self-soothe until they are a few months old. If she's crying, try to address her needs right away, and she will likely be calmer overall. Sleep training is not recommended until your baby reaches 4-6 months.

Just keep in mind that giving birth is a major event. Between recovery, changing hormones levels, and getting used to carrying for your new little one, it's okay to feel a bit overwhelmed! You may even find yourself crying for no reason as your hormones return to a normal level. Be patient, take care of yourself, don't be afraid to accept and ask for help, and enjoy every moment with your little baby! This moment won't last forever.

Additional Resources

If you are preparing for childbirth, check out this article for a comprehensive list of things to try, including diet, exercise, stretches, meditation, chiropractic, and more.

Read or listen to my positive first birth story.

Learn more about the "wonder weeks," or your child's developmental spurts and how to help her through them.

Learn more about baby "language."

Postpartum Depression and Self-Care

Postpartum depression can take a serious toll on your overall health following childbirth. As your body returns to its pre-pregnancy state, your hormones change. While mood swings and mild emotional changes are normal during and after pregnancy, some people have a much more extreme experience. If you think you have postpartum depression, speak with your doctor. He/she can provide tailored advice and may suggest medication. Depression does not mean there is something wrong with you, and you will feel yourself again soon enough! I know it's tough, but hang in there, mama!

Just remember to be gentle with yourself. Your sleep isn't ideal, your independence has all but disappeared, and your body is changing. It's okay to feel low. Be gentle with your feelings. Take your mental health seriously. Your experience is real and valid. Remember that you have needs, too. Don't be afraid to reach out for help. I had a hard time asking for help because I believed I should be able to handle everything on my own. Next time I will be much more accepting of assistance!

Here are some tips to help you cope with these changes:

- Just breathe. Practicing deep, mindful breaths is an excellent way to calm your mind and body. Be patient. It will get better, I promise!

- Be grateful. Keep a simple gratitude journal that you update each night.

- Look outside yourself. Who do you know who may be struggling more than you? What can you do to help them?

- Talk with someone. Speak with a loved one, a doctor, a counselor, etc. Sometimes just writing your thoughts, feelings, and experiences or saying them out loud can shed a new positive light on things.

- Make time for yourself. I know this is hard when your little one needs you 24/7. But if you can even take a few minutes to read, color, take a warm bath, or just lay down and breathe while he/she is sleeping, it can do wonders for your mental health!

Making Time for Self-Care

I didn't experience postpartum depression with my infant, but I honestly believe I experienced it when I first assumed full-time care for my stepdaughter. Suddenly, I was thrust from complete independence to complete responsibility for another little human being. She was in kindergarten at the time, so you would think that I'd be just fine with the hours she was away from home. But it was still hard.

The first time she was home for two weeks straight was Christmas break. And I completely lost it. Nonstop caring for her needs, being there for her emotionally, answering her questions, playing with her, and focusing all my attention on her was a lot to take on all at once. Where before I enjoyed at least my mental space, now *everything* I had was going to her.

I remember waking up each morning with the most horrible sense of dread. I couldn't stand the thought of enduring yet another day. I knew this one would be just as hard as the last. And the worst part? I did not have the option to stop, take a breather, and take a different route. My child would have needs, regardless of my mental state.

I have always wanted to be a mom. As a teenager, I imagined myself playing with my future kids, teaching them, loving them, and always being there for them. I just assumed that once the time came, I would find all my joy in them. I wouldn't need anything else.

Turns out, having a baby, or adopting, or marrying someone with children is a *huge* change. We don't have the option to take on the new responsibility gradually. Of course, we love our kids, and we love spending time with them, but our minds and bodies are not always ready for the change!

You Don't Have to Do It All on Your Own

I continued to struggle as a new parent until I allowed myself to believe that I had needs, too. Initially, I honestly believed that I could and *should* be doing everything myself. Afterall, I was a mom, so I should be able to take on the full weight of parenthood. It was my duty.

However, the reality is that our needs do not disappear after we have a child. Our minds and bodies still require care if we are to be fully present for our families. Neglecting our needs only makes it harder to care for the needs of others.

Have you ever been on an airplane? What instructions do they give you regarding oxygen masks?

Put on *your* oxygen mask *before* attempting to help someone with theirs.

Why? Because if you don't put your mask on, and you run out of oxygen, *you ain't helping nobody!*

The same thing applies to motherhood! If you are not taking care of your needs, you cannot take care of anyone else's needs either! It simply doesn't work.

For me, one of the most basic needs to address was taking time for myself. My physical health was pretty good, but my mental health was crumbling.

During that challenging Christmas break, my spouse saw the struggle and encouraged me to take a break. While he was with his daughter, I had a moment to think about my needs. A simple walk around the neighborhood was so therapeutic and needed.

So how do I ease the transition?

A few months into motherhood, I started working on some of my hobbies again. I finished up a book I'd been writing, I added to my blog, I started learning videography and film editing. And suddenly, each time I woke up in the morning, I was excited to meet the new day! No longer did I dread the coming routine. Instead, I couldn't wait to get started! I knew there was so much to do, so much to learn, so many new things to try.

My family is 100% my priority, and I love spending time with them. Taking a moment each day to learn something new or do something I love breathes life back into me that I can share with them!

Whatever your interests are, take some time to write them down. Include anything that helps you relax and feel great. Here are some suggestions:

- Take a warm bath with your favorite bath salts and music.
- Snuggle up under your favorite blanket and read a good book.
- Go for a drive.
- Go for a walk around the neighborhood or a local park.
- Peruse your favorite craft store for inspiration.

- Learn a new skill on YouTube.
- Make a craft for your baby.
- Make a fun craft with your older kids.
- Write in your journal. Or write your thoughts and feelings on a paper that you can tear up or burn (surprisingly therapeutic!).
- Join a group yoga class or other exercise class.
- Color, draw, or paint.
- Make a paper mâché piñata.

You may find that many of the things you enjoy can be done for or with your family. Personal development and learning can be highly therapeutic. It gives you an immediate sense of accomplishment.

Find Joy in the Small Wins

Parenting often yields slow, long-term rewards because the growth of your child and your relationships is gradual. Sometimes it's nice to work on a project where the outcomes are within your control. For example, if you are making a quilt, it is easy to see the project progress. Each time you sew a new piece on, the quilt grows. You have control over how quickly it grows and get to learn along the way.

In reality, parenting isn't much different. Though the long-term outcomes of our efforts are largely out of our control, we can find joy and satisfaction in the short-term wins. For example, watching your baby smile for the first time is incredibly rewarding and makes all the sleepless nights inconsequential. And then her first laugh, and her first step, and her first words. It all fills you up with joy and love for your little one!

If you have older children, you know that focusing on these small wins is vital during the tougher teaching moments. When your child is learning to read, it may feel painfully slow at first. You may wonder if your child is learning as fast as other children. But focusing on the fact that he is not yet reading chapter books only increases his and your sense of discouragement.

However, every time he learns a new word or sound combination, that's a small win! It doesn't matter how quickly he learns new sounds. What matters is that he is learning!

Tougher yet is teaching unmeasurable skills such as patience, listening, and honesty. It can be incredibly difficult to notice the small steps your child is making towards healthier habits and attitudes. But do your best to notice them none-the-less.

In this stage, don't forget to take time for yourself. As I stated previously, taking time to do something you love can help you relax and have more emotional energy to be present with your children. Your children need *you* more than anything else right now. They have big emotions, too, and will watch how you handle yours. If you take the time to breathe, re-collect yourself, and take breaks, your kids will learn healthy and positive ways to handle big feelings.

No journey is perfect, and every child is different. We all have different needs, but we all share the need to be loved. I know you love your baby, your kids, and your family more than words can express. Don't forget to love yourself!

And don't forget to get your free workbook/journal to help with your journey to better health!

SCAN WITH YOUR CAMERA TO GET YOUR WORKBOOK!

Day 1: Affirmations for Self-Care

It's time to start your 30-day journey to better health! Are you excited?

The mind has a powerful effect on the body. While the brain sends and interprets signals to regulate your body, even your thoughts, emotions, and experiences have a profound impact on your health. Even if you develop a strict workout routine and start eating plenty of nutritious foods, you're quite likely to slip back into old habits if the issue isn't taken up by the roots.

Have you ever seen a plate of cookies on your kitchen counter and forbidden yourself from eating them? What happened as soon as you told yourself you couldn't have those cookies? You probably couldn't stop thinking about them, right? Your mind acted out in protest, and you might have even felt hungrier until you finally gave in and grabbed a cookie. The mind is a powerful tool, and we can use that to our advantage!

We will address several ways the mind affects the body throughout this entire book. In general, our goal is to develop a shift in your mindset. By the end of these thirty days, I hope you see your health in a more positive light and genuinely enjoy caring for your body. Exercise and nutritious eating are invigorating and fun! Change is exciting! Learning is energizing!

Focusing on what you want to change can make it much harder to change. For example, I've noticed that when I stress about my weight, I gain more weight. But when I accept my body and make peace with how I look right now, I start to lose weight without even trying. I've also noticed that when I constantly remind myself how tired I am, I feel so much more tired. But on days where I don't have time to think about how exhausted I am, I do quite well. Instead, telling myself that I have ample energy fuels me both mentally and physically.

It is so important to remember that you are what you believe you are. If you tell yourself that you are weak, unhealthy, and incapable, that's exactly how you will act. However, if you tell yourself that you are strong, healthy, and capable, you will make decisions that draw you closer to those ideals. And there have been plenty of studies to demonstrate the effect of positive thinking on health.

Each day throughout the 30 days, you will be given a positive affirmation to repeat to yourself. After reading the challenge for the day, look yourself in the mirror, and recite the affirmation. Throughout the day, repeat the affirmation in your mind. Replace negative thoughts with this one positive affirmation.

You may not believe every affirmation. Some of them may not yet be a reality for you. However, as you repeat these affirmations, you will begin to believe them and start to *make* them a reality.

Make sure to say each affirmation out loud. When I'm in the car alone and thinking over a bad feeling or memory, I can say aloud that I am a good person and that I am capable and loved, and it has a huge impact on my conviction. Do the same! Say it loud and clear, "I am capable! I am healthy and strong! I have energy! I am beautiful and worthy! I am good at making healthy changes and developing healthy habits!" Say it until you believe it!

Today you have a list of affirmations to read and practice. Anytime you start to stress about your weight or your body image, read and repeat these affirmations.

I am comfortable in my body.

I am grateful for all my body is capable of.

My mind is strong.

My mind is at peace.

I am confident in my ability to change.

I am at peace with where I'm at right now.

I love to live and learn.

I am ready and excited to make healthy changes in my life.

I feel good when I take care of my body.

I enjoy finding healthy foods to eat.

My health is important to me. This is a time commitment I am willing to make.

I love being a mom and find joy in caring for my newborn. I can provide the love, care, and support she/he needs.

I have ample resources to share with loved ones. I have time, energy, and confidence to be there for my child.

Notes:

_____

_____

_____

_____

_____

_____

_____

_____

_____

_____

_____

_____

_____

_____

_____

_____

Day 2: Should I Diet?

First thing to note is that with just about any diet, you can successfully lose weight, as long as you are willing to *stick with that diet*. The problem is that "diets" are usually temporary, and often difficult to follow for an extended period. They may be time consumptive, labor intensive, or leave you feeling hungry all the time. And when you finally give up and return to your normal eating patterns, whatever weight you just lost comes running back.

Real weight loss comes from *real* lasting change. It comes as you gradually make small, permanent lifestyle changes.

Here are some characteristics of a good "diet."

- Sustainable
- Not restrictive
- Not time consuming
- Not expensive, requiring you to buy unusual products

- Not encouraging excessive consumption of one food or food group
- Well balanced between food groups
- Nutrient dense and satisfying
- Keeps you full between meals
- Permanent, not temporary

Keep in mind that the goal of dieting should be to promote overall health, not just one health outcome. For example, the Keto diet is designed to help you lose weight, while the Paleo diet is meant to reduce inflammation in the body. And the guidelines from each of these diets are very different. While the Keto diet recommends avoiding tropical fruits, the Paleo diet raves over their health benefits. You may hear that bananas are bad for weight loss due to their high carb content. However, bananas are also rich in nutrients and fibers that may reduce the risk of cancer and chronic disease.

Remember. What may be good for weight loss may not be good for your heart, gut, brain, etc.

Another important thing to note is that healthy weight loss does not occur right away. Generally, your body composition changes first. You will start to develop more muscle as you lose fat. Since muscle weighs more than fat, your scale may not reflect the healthy changes occurring in your body. If you lose a ton of weight right away after starting a diet, the cause is most likely water loss. Dramatically reducing your carb intake causes an especially substantial reduction in body water. While this water loss is not generally harmful, it is not the same as fat reduction and does not reflect healthy weight loss.

Today's challenge is to think of one small change you would like to make today. Write it down, tape it to your fridge, share it with your family, and then take action to implement the change.

For example, one simple thing you can do is find the candy drawer and empty it out. But don't just leave it empty! These drawers tend to refill themselves! Instead, go out and find some healthier snacks to take their place: your favorite granola bars, nuts and seeds, whole grain crackers, dried fruit, protein bites, popcorn, etc. Try to find things you enjoy!

I love making food replacements. Telling myself that I can't have ice cream anymore, for example, is really challenging. The more I limit my intake, the more I want that ice cream. And usually, after a while of mourning my loss, I snap and eat a whole bunch of ice cream at once.

In addition, restricting intake can actually *cause* overeating. Imagine one of your favorite treats sitting on the counter, in my case, the ice cream, just waiting for you to dip a spoon in it. But you are, quote, "on a diet," so you can't eat that ice cream. It's forbidden. So, you return it to the freezer for your spouse or roommate to eat instead. And then you leave for work or go about your day.

But you still want that ice cream, and you're struggling to keep it off your mind. To curb the craving, you find an apple and eat it. But that really doesn't satisfy. It's just not ice cream. So, still hungry, you pull a granola bar from your bag. And then you take a trip to the vending machine. By this point, you're not really hungry, at least not physically, but your brain is still telling you that you are hungry because you're not giving it the one thing it wants. Finally, you return home and open the freezer. The ice cream is still sitting there, and you think, "you know what, I've had a long day. I deserve some ice cream." So, you pull it out, serve yourself a generous scoop, and happily wolf it down, satisfied at last. Sound familiar?

Now, if you really are committed to cutting ice cream out of your diet, at some point you're not going to crave ice cream anymore. However, this can take weeks and is challenging. A great way to start weeding out the nutritionally poor foods from your diet is to make small substitutions. Don't substitute salad for ice cream. Believe me, it won't satisfy. No matter how many times you tell yourself that you are eating ice cream, it's just not ice cream. It's salad.

Buuuuut, if you can start by simply finding a healthier ice cream, that's a great step in the right direction! There are lots of products out there with lower sugar contents, higher protein, and less artificial ingredients or preservatives. Keep your eyes open and get excited to explore new options.

Then the next step? Try switching from your healthier ice-cream to yogurt with sliced fruit on top. See where this is going?

I had to cut dairy out of my diet in my mid-twenties, and making the switch was challenging at first. One thing I struggled to avoid was milk chocolate. However, I found that I really enjoyed dark chocolate and gradually increased the cocoa percentage until I was regularly enjoying 85% dark chocolate. My favorite brand has very little sugar and surprisingly high levels of iron and fiber! Now, anything sweeter than 85% isn't palatable to me. The point is, that small dietary changes *do* affect your cravings and your affinity towards certain foods. It is entirely possible to rid your house of unhealthy foods, but doing so gradually will greatly increase your chances of success.

Again, the challenge for today is to think of one *small* change you would like to make today. Write it down, tape it to your fridge, share it with your family, and then take action to implement the change.

Notes:

_____

_____

_____

_____

_____

_____

_____

_____

_____

_____

_____

_____

_____

_____

_____

_____

Day 3: Start with Micro Habits

Daily affirmation: I feel good when I fuel my body well.

Going from zero to 100 can be incredibly difficult and is rarely sustainable. How many times have you decided to eat better or exercise more and have quit before the end of the month? Why is it so hard to develop lasting changes?

There are a couple of important reasons to discuss: for one, each of us has a "threshold of success," and secondly, we overlook the power of micro habits.

Threshold of Success

Sometimes we fear success; we unknowingly limit ourselves, because where we are at *now* is familiar territory. We see a little success then suddenly fall back, uncomfortable and unwilling to continue. This is where we hit our "threshold of success." We recognize that eating nutritious foods and exercising daily will be both joyful and energizing.

However, we identify with our current weight and habits and have a hard time visualizing anything different.

Learn to love and embrace change. Before anything can improve, you'll need to decide to not stay where you are.

The Power of Micro Habits

We all want to be lean, fit, and healthy as soon as possible, right? The trouble is, every time we start going to the gym or cut out dessert, the habit fails to stick, and we find ourselves back at square one. The reality is that it is much, *much* easier to create lasting habits if we start very, very small. But often we overlook these tiny changes, because they don't quickly produce the results we seek.

The irony is, that we'd probably reach our goals a lot faster by sticking with these small, micro habits than by chasing the grander lifestyle changes. Why? Because we can realistically and permanently develop micro habits and then slowly build on them.

Let me explain with an example. Say you want to eat less sugar. You can go cold turkey and get rid of all the junk food in your house, but the reality is that your mind and body are not ready for the change. The next time you walk by the candy aisle or attend a party, those sweets will still be calling your name! Instead, you can try first developing a micro habit. Perhaps every time you reach for a soda or a treat, you decide to drink a full glass of water first. You keep doing this every day for a whole month, until it just becomes second nature to drink water before consuming something sweet. Then, for the next month, each time you want to eat a treat, you drink your glass of water, *and* eat a handful of roasted almonds. Then the next month, you start cutting the treat in half and tossing the other half. As these little habits start to become second nature, you make new associations with your actions. Initially, your brain connected sweets with pleasure. But now, you are beginning to enjoy the water and almonds and the satisfaction your stomach feels. You start to recognize your cravings for sweets as your body's need for nourishment.

Here is a short list of micro habits you can start to implement. Pick just two or three of these habits to work on at a time and stick with them for a month before building on them. You want to pick habits that are simple and easy to accomplish each day.

- Brush your teeth right after dinner
- Drink a full glass of water when you wake up
- Eat eggs or nuts with your breakfast
- Write down one thing you are grateful for at the end of the day
- Stretch for 1 minute when you wake up or before bed
- Smile at yourself in the mirror or while driving to work

Notes:

_____

_____

_____

_____

_____

_____

_____

Day 4: Cardio Vs Strength Training

Shortly after giving birth, it's not a good idea to return to vigorous workouts right away. Make sure to follow the advice of your doctor or OB-GYN, who will examine you and let you know when it's okay to resume regular exercises. Generally, after six weeks you will be allowed to return to your full workout routine.

Have you ever wondered what the best type of exercise is for weight loss? Have you considered that one type may be more effective than another?

There are two types of exercise: aerobic, and anaerobic, which basically translate to cardio and muscle exercises. Aerobic, or cardio exercises, utilize oxygen and generally involve longer periods of moderate activity, such as walking or jogging. Anaerobic exercises require short, intense bursts of activity that don't utilize oxygen. Examples are weightlifting and HIIT (high-intensity-interval-training), which we will discuss later in the month.

While cardio exercises are great for your heart and your overall health, they're not necessarily great for weight loss. They do burn energy, or calories, in the moment, but their overall effect on metabolism is minimal. In addition, cardio exercises tend to sap a lot of glucose (sugar) from the bloodstream, leaving you quite hungry afterwards. When you eat a meal to satisfy that hunger, you're essentially netting zero—replacing all the calories you just burned off.

Anaerobic exercises, on the other hand, have the wonderful tendency to keep burning fat, even *after* you've completed the exercise. They build muscle, boost your metabolism, and don't require as much of a time commitment to produce results. I once knew someone with a lot of obvious muscle mass. He wasn't a bodybuilder, per se, but you could tell he loved the gym. When I asked him how long he had to exercise each day to stay so fit, his response was, "Ten minutes." Ten minutes! If I told you that you could work out for just 10 minutes a day and get in great shape, would you do it? I think so! That's something you could totally do while baby is napping or spending time with Dad! It's all about exercising the right way.

But, just to be clear, I'm not suggesting you ditch your morning walk or evening jog. These movements are still great for your heart health, and even just being outside for a bit has great physical and emotional benefits. However, if you are looking for a more efficient way to burn fat and lose weight, anaerobic exercises are your best option.

Remember, one of the biggest keys to weight loss is boosting your metabolism and limiting hunger so you don't feel like you are starving all the time. More muscle means a quicker metabolism.

Today's challenge is your first strength workout. The next few exercises will be as follows: cardio, upper body and core, HIIT, yoga, lower body ladders, and upper body ladders. All of these workouts (except for some of the upper body exercises) are body weight only, so they don't require any equipment other than your shoes. But, of course, you can always add a pair of dumbbells or ankle weights to add resistance!

Don't know what at-home workout equipment to collect? There are so many different products designed for use at home, but is any of it really necessary? I've outlined a list of equipment I like to use at home that is inexpensive and easy to use. Access the article here to start building your DIY home gym.

Lower body workout

Make sure to breathe through each exercise. Holding your breath during strength workouts may be tempting. Instead, inhale, then exhale on the lift. During pulses, just breathe evenly. Exercises are illustrated at the end of the chapter.

Find a timer you can set up in front of you to keep track of each interval. You can also use your phone or a watch or simply count in your head.

20 curtsy lunges, alternating right and left legs (1)

Curtsy lunge on right leg: pulse for 20 seconds

Curtsy lunge on left leg: pulse for 20 seconds

30 calf raises (2)

15 sumo squats, then pulse for 30 seconds (3)

20 chair squats (feet together), then pulse for 15 seconds (4)

20 fire-hydrants on each leg: on all fours, keep your right leg bent at a 90-degree angle as you raise it to the right 20 times. Repeat with left leg. (5)

20 standing back-leg lifts: stand on your left leg and raise your right leg straight backwards, maintaining only a slight bend in the knee. Focus on tightening your glutes. Repeat 20 times with your right leg and then with your left leg. (6)

Repeat workout one or two more times.

Stretch

As you stretch, make sure to breathe in before stretching, then breathe out as you deepen each stretch. Rather than counting the seconds for each stretch, you can count your breaths. I like to hold each stretch for four deep breaths.

Hamstring stretch: stand on left foot, using a wall or chair for support if needed. Bend right leg and grab your foot with your right hand. Pull gently to feel a stretch on the front of your thigh. Hold for 15 seconds and repeat on the left side. (7)

Next, sit on the floor and spread your legs wide. Reach to the right, keeping your foot flexed, for 15 seconds. Repeat on the left side. (8)

Bring your feet together with your legs straight out in front of you. Reach forward to again feel a stretch along the backs of your legs. Hold for 15 seconds. (9)

Pull your feet towards you for a butterfly stretch. Lean forward until you can feel a stretch in your inner thighs. Hold for 15 seconds. (10)

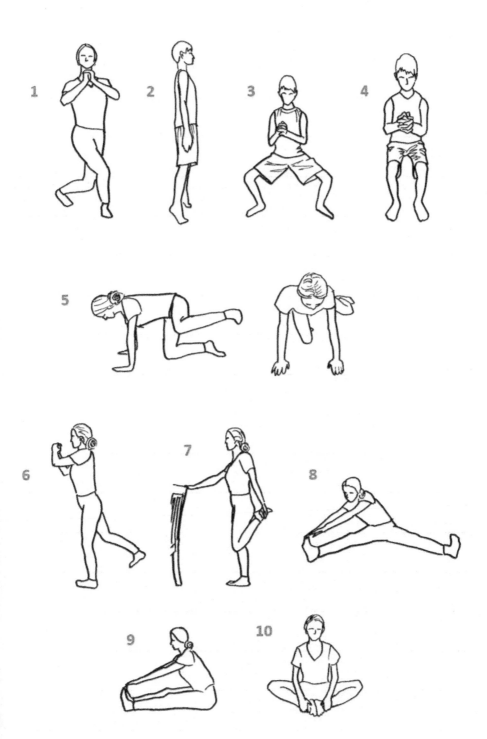

Notes:

_____

_____

_____

_____

_____

_____

_____

_____

_____

_____

_____

_____

_____

_____

Day 5: What is Homeostasis?

Daily affirmation: My body is designed to work with me, not against me. I make healthy choices to support my body and give it what it needs to thrive.

Throughout my schooling, I was largely taught that as long as calories consumed are less than calories burned, then you will lose weight. While this is generally true, there are some very important pieces missing from this puzzle. For starters, plenty of people have tried the calorie counting method and failed because it is time consuming, for one, and you are constantly hungry due to the calorie deficit.

Secondly, this idea is way over-simplified.

Your body likes to maintain something called *homeostasis*, which keeps your health and your systems working in a regular and consistent pattern. Homeostasis is a state of equilibrium. One example is your body temperature. Your body is very good at maintaining a body temperature of about 97.6 degrees F. Very rarely does your temperature fluctuate above or below, and when it does, it suggests a problem.

The same goes for your body weight. When you eat a larger meal than normal, your body makes necessary adjustments, so all that food doesn't go immediately to your waistline. For one, you feel full, and your metabolism picks up a bit to process the excess food. And the same goes for undereating. When you consume less calories than you are expending, your body responds by sending out hunger signals and slowing your metabolism. This is why it can be so hard to lose weight. Your body will literally sabotage your efforts because it thinks you are starving yourself!

Of course, if you continue to eat excessively, you will begin to gain weight over time. Likewise, if you continue to restrict your calories, you will eventually lose weight. However, you usually have to consume less and less to make up for the adjustments your body is making. Calorie restriction alone is not enough to help you lose weight.

So how, then, do you lose weight? The trick lies in eating and exercising in such a way that speeds up your metabolism (doesn't slow it down) and doesn't leave you starving. As we will discuss later, it's important to eat balanced meals with good sources of protein, healthy fats, and fibers. And completing exercises that strengthen your muscles is great for boosting your metabolism.

Now that you've learned a little about homeostasis, pull out your journal and write down what you've learned.

Today's challenge is to make a home-cooked meal. Aim to include a vegetable, a whole grain, and a protein, and enjoy some fresh fruit for dessert. Here are a few meal suggestions:

- Stir-fry with bell pepper, broccoli, carrots, and diced chicken. Serve over brown rice. Enjoy mango slices for dessert.

- Turkey sandwiches on whole-wheat bread with lettuce and tomato. Enjoy strawberries and blueberries for dessert.

- Three-bean vegan chili. Beans fall into both the protein category and the vegetable category. They are also a great source of fiber and healthy carbs, so you do not need to include a grain with this meal. However, you could serve whole-grain cornbread on the side if desired. Enjoy raspberries and blackberries or apple slices for dessert.

Meal planning can be super overwhelming. Believe me, I know. As a mom of two little girls, I have a hard time finding a spare moment to prepare a meal. My 7-month-old always wants to be held, which makes it way harder to get anything done. Plus, after the meal is prepared, I have all the dishes to get done! When I was on my own, I absolutely loved cooking. Now, it is overwhelming just thinking about it.

It does help a TON to have a simple meal plan ahead of time. I love using a meal planning app called Whisk, which really simplifies the planning and auto-generates a shopping list for you.

Notes:

_____

_____

_____

_____

_____

_____

Day 6: Turkey, Bacon, Avocado Sandwich

Daily affirmation: I love trying new, delicious, nutritious foods!

I love making turkey, bacon, avocado sandwiches, because they're super quick and easy, packed with protein and healthy fats, and very satisfying. Make sure to adjust the recipe size according to your needs! You may feel quite full after only half a sandwich.

After Thanksgiving, you can use your leftover turkey to fill the sandwich, or throughout the year, use a good-quality deli turkey. I prefer to go to the deli counter at the grocery store and get freshly sliced meats rather than purchasing pre-sliced turkey. The texture of freshly sliced meats is better for this recipe. I also prefer turkey bacon over regular bacon, since it is lower in saturated fat. However, you can use regular bacon if you prefer.

If you want to reduce the carbs in this recipe, try making your sandwich open-faced, or remove the bread all together. You can chop up the turkey, bacon, and avocado, and stir it together with a little salt, pepper, mayo, and lemon juice for a delicious, low-carb variation.

40

Ingredients:

1 tbsp mayonnaise
1 tsp lemon juice
2 slices whole-grain or gluten-free bread, toasted
2 slices turkey meat
2 strips turkey bacon, cooked
2 thin circular slices granny smith apple
½ avocado, sliced
Salt and pepper to taste

Directions:

Combine mayonnaise and lemon juice. Spread on both slices of toasted bread. Layer turkey, bacon, apple slices, and avocado in between the two slices. Sprinkle salt and pepper on the avocado slices. Enjoy!

Notes:

_____

_____

_____

_____

_____

_____

_____

Turkey Bacon Avocado Sandwich

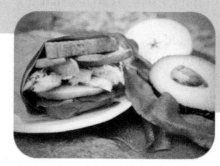

Serving size: 1
Calories: 505

Prep time: 10 min
Cooking time: 5 min

Ingredients

1 tbsp mayonnaise
1 tsp lemon juice
2 slices whole grain bread
toasted
2 slices turkey meat
2 strips cooked bacon
2 thin circular slices of
granny smith apple
½ avocado *sliced*
Salt and pepper *to taste*

Directions

1. Combine mayonnaise and lemon juice. Spread on both slices of toasted bread.

2. Layer turkey, bacon, apple slices, and avocado on bread.

3. Add salt and pepper to taste. Enjoy!

21g
30g
43g
10g
14g

Day 7: Cardio Workout

Daily affirmation: I have ample energy to thrive throughout my day.

Previously, we discussed that cardio, or aerobic, exercises are generally moderate intensity and involve the consumption of oxygen by the body. A great cardio exercise you can do without much thought is simply taking a run-walk around the neighborhood. Try running in intervals. For example, run or jog for 2 minutes, then walk for 1 minute. As your stamina increases, you will be able to run for longer intervals and take shorter breaks.

There are also many stationary exercises you can do to get your heart pumping. Examples include jumping jacks, lateral jumps, burpees, jogging in place, high knees, squat jumps, mountain climbers, and butt kicks. Many stationary exercises heavily target your muscles as well as you heart. Make sure to maintain a good posture and keep your core tight (abs firm) to protect your back and improve the quality of your workout.

Today's workout is a series of exercises that can be done in your home. So, grab your water bottle, some tennis shoes, and find a spot with a bit of space to exercise. The whole workout takes about 16 minutes, but you may repeat it as you wish. Let's begin!

Warm up (2:30)

30 sec arm circles forward (1)

30 sec arm circles backward

15 sec swing arms back, then forward and around opposite shoulders, like you are giving yourself repeated hugs (2)

30 sec jog in place

15 sec stand with legs wide apart and slowly reach down to touch the ground (3)

15 sec reach over to right leg (4)

15 sec reach over to left leg

Workout (10:40)

60 sec jumping jacks

20 sec rest

60 sec jumping jacks

20 sec rest

60 sec butt-kicks (jog in place, but your heels should hit your butt)

20 sec rest

60 sec butt-kicks

20 sec rest

60 sec skaters (lateral jumps) (5)

20 sec rest

60 sec skaters (lateral jumps)

     20 sec rest

60 sec jump forward three times, then jog backwards

     20 sec rest

60 sec jump forward three times, then jog backwards

     20 sec rest

Cool down and stretch (2:40)

45 sec walk in place

15 sec stand on left foot. Lift right foot and grab with right hand. Pull foot gently towards your body to stretch front of thigh. If needed, place left hand on wall or chair for balance. Repeat on right foot. (6)

10 sec stretch right arm across your chest (7)

10 sec stretch right arm behind your back (8)

10 sec stretch left arm across your chest

10 sec stretch left arm behind your back

Sit down with legs spread wide (9)

15 sec reach towards your right foot

15 sec reach towards your left foot

Pull legs together, straight out in front of you (10)

15 sec reach towards your toes, pulling your toes towards your fingers to stretch the calves

Notes:

_____

_____

_____

_____

_____

_____

_____

_____

_____

_____

_____

_____

_____

_____

_____

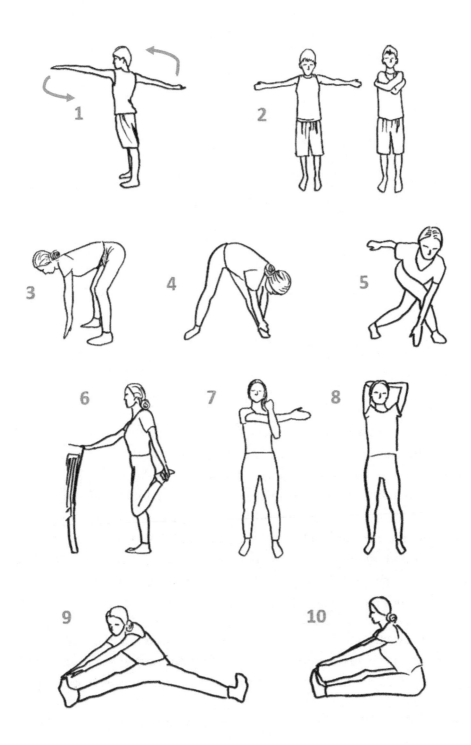

Day 8: Integrate, Integrate, Integrate

Daily affirmation: I have time and energy to make healthy changes in my life.

One of the biggest reasons diets fail is because they quickly become impractical or time consuming. When the necessities of daily life start to take over, the diet drops to the side. Sure, if you have nothing but time on your hands and a budget to support whatever foods and supplements suit your fancy, you can diet all you want! I can tell you though, I've never found such time to be so readily available. As a student, I was busy working and studying. As a mom, I'm always busy cleaning, teaching, changing diapers, bouncing my baby to sleep, cooking, and you know…other mom things. There's never enough time in the day!

So how exactly are you supposed to find the time and energy to home cook all your meals, portion out snacks for your pantry, exercise, explore new recipes, learn about your health, and implement necessary changes?

First of all, I very much believe that you can make time for anything you truly consider a priority. However, there *is* a way to make lifestyle changes much simpler and easier. It's called *integrating*.

For example: when my first baby was born, she never wanted to be set down. If I wasn't feeding her, I was bouncing or holding her, and the only way I could get anything done was by letting someone else hold her for a turn.

This trend continued for several weeks, months even. It was nearly impossible to exercise. Eventually, I started doing gentle lower-body exercises with her in my arms, simply in an effort to bounce her to sleep or comfort her. I found that she liked the movements, and my muscles liked the work. In addition to taking walks around the neighborhood with her in the baby carrier or stroller, these leg exercises became my daily workout routine.

During college, exercising was great for de-stressing physically, but didn't much help me decompress mentally. So, when I really needed a break from all the working and studying, I would take my tablet to the gym, prop it up on an elliptical, and watch my favorite movie or tv show while exercising. Or I would listen to an audio book. By the end, I felt great: energized, rejuvenated, and strong. It was the perfect combination for me.

You've undoubtedly found ways to maximize your time already. So how can you do so with your healthy lifestyle changes? What are you already doing that you can simply modify to meet your goals? What can you replace? What things are you doing that are unnecessary or even damaging to your physical and mental health?

A Few Ways to Integrate Healthy Habits

Exercise with your kids: take them for a walk around the park, do jumping jacks, go outside, etc.

Get your family involved. If you are already eating dinner together, why not make it together? And when you go grocery shopping, try taking them along to pick out their favorite fruits and vegetables, and get them excited about trying new, nutritious foods and snacks.

Watch your favorite TV show on the treadmill.

During your weekly planning, quickly jot down 3-5 healthy meals you'd like to prepare. If you have the Whisk app, you can very easily create a meal plan for the week and add the ingredients directly to your shopping list. It takes maybe five minutes for me to create my meal plan each week (unless I get caught up looking at all the delicious recipes!). And five minutes is easy to find.

Get creative. Pick a healthy habit and write down how you will integrate it into your life today.

Notes:

_____

_____

_____

_____

_____

_____

_____

_____

Day 9: Well-Balanced Smoothies

Daily affirmation: I am energized by uplifting human interactions. I emanate a positive energy that uplifts those around me.

Have you ever considered how much sugar you are consuming from all that blended up fruit in a smoothie? Sure, you're getting a healthy dose of vitamins and minerals, but when you blend up fruits, you break apart the complex structure of carbohydrates and fibers that generally slows digestion. When you eat a whole fruit, those structures remain intact, thus slowing the entrance of sugar into your bloodstream.

But, smoothie lovers, don't you worry! There is a way to improve the balance of your smoothies and fit them into your healthy lifestyle.

Here are a couple of my favorite smoothie recipes that balance sugars, proteins, healthy fats, and fibers quite well!

Notes:

_____

_____

_____

_____

_____

_____

_____

_____

_____

_____

_____

_____

_____

_____

_____

_____

Choco-Avo-Banana Smoothie

Ingredients

1 banana, ripe
½ avocado
1 tbsp cocoa powder
1 tbsp peanut butter
1 tsp vanilla extract
1 cup milk of choice (I use unsweetened almond milk)

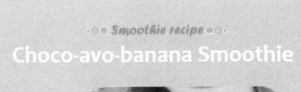

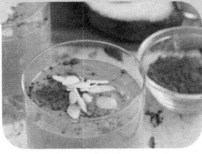

Serving size: 1
Calories: 340

Prep time: 5 min
Cooking time: N/A

Ingredients

1 banana *ripe*
½ avocado
1 tbsp cocoa powder
1 tbsp peanut butter
1 tsp vanilla extract
1 cup milk of choice *I use unsweetened almond milk*

Directions

Combine all ingredients in a blender and blend until smooth.

Enjoy!

8g
20g
40g
9g
17g

Very Berry Smoothie

Ingredients

¼ cup raspberries
¼ cup blueberries
¼ cup strawberries
¼ cup blackberries
¼ cup oats
1 tbsp chia seeds or ground flax seeds
1 cup unsweetened coconut milk (not the canned kind)
1 tsp vanilla extract

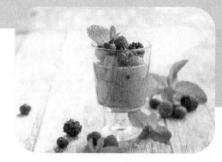

● ● ● *Smoothie recipe* ● ● ●

Very Berry Smoothie

Serving size: 1
Calories: 304

Prep time: 5 min
Cooking time: N/A

Ingredients

Directions

¼ cup raspberries
¼ cup blueberries
¼ cup strawberries
¼ cup blackberries
¼ cup oats
1 tbsp chia seeds or
ground flax seeds
1 cup coconut milk *not
the canned kind*
1 tsp vanilla extract

Combine all ingredients in a
blender and blend until
smooth.

Enjoy!

10g
14g
46g
13g
9g

Day 10: Upper Body and Core Workout

Strengthening the core can help reduce back pain and improve posture. A strong core is also really important for maintaining balance and stability in other exercises such as yoga and dance aerobics. Today, you will be working muscles in your back, shoulders, abs, biceps, and triceps. You can complete your workout with a short walk or jog to get your blood flowing!

Diastasis Recti and Pelvic Floor

Diastasis recti is the parting of the abdominal wall during pregnancy. After childbirth, it is wise to avoid certain core exercises, which can actually make the split worse. Split abs can cause instability and back pain. During the first six weeks, engage in simple core exercises such as:

- Cat/cows (pelvic tilts)
- Toe touches
- Modified planks and side planks

Some exercises and daily movements can make diastasis recti worse. Try to avoid the following:

- Overarching your lower back (one way or the other) or slouching. It is important to maintain a neutral spine at all times.

- Bending over at the waist to pick up your baby or other items. Instead, bend your knees.

- Crunches or similar core exercises.

It is also important to strengthen your pelvic floor muscles through Kegel exercises. This helps prevent wetting yourself every time you jump or cough. To practice Kegel exercises, contract the muscles you use to stop the flow of urine. You can find these muscles while using the bathroom by starting and stopping the flow of urine repeatedly. While you are in the car on your way to work, watching a movie, etc., tighten these muscles slowly for ten seconds, hold for ten seconds, then release for ten seconds. Do this 10-20 times daily. You can also practice Kegel exercises with your core exercises.

Once your doctor or OB-GYN gives you the go-ahead to resume regular core exercises, you no longer need to modify your routine for diastasis recti.

Warm up:

Arm circles forward 10 times

Arm circles backward 10 times

Arm swings in front and across your body 10 times

Workout:

Complete each exercise, take a 20 second break, then repeat. Make sure to stretch after the workout.

15 pushups (on your toes or on your knees) (1)

15 triceps dips (2)

45 second hold plank position (3)

20 Russian twists (4)

10 pike pushups (5)

20 bicycle crunches (6)

20 supermans (7)

20 bicep curls with weight of choice (8)

Notes:

_____

_____

_____

_____

_____

_____

_____

_____

_____

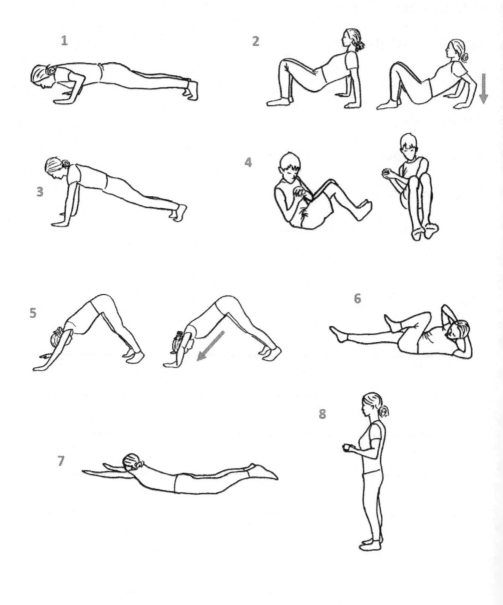

Day 11: What Motivates You?

Everyone is motivated by something, good or bad. What motivates you?

What makes you get up in the morning? Are you motivated simply by necessity? Are you excited to get out of bed?

What are your passions? What makes you forget to eat and keeps you up at odd hours? What are you so excited to do each day that you jump out of bed in the morning and can hardly dress yourself for fear of wasting precious time?

Take a moment now to stop reading and write down all your thoughts! Really dig in deep.

Now consider how all this relates to weight loss. Why do you want to lose weight? Is it because you want to look thinner? Is it because you want to be around long enough to enjoy your grandchildren? Do you want to have more energy to pursue hobbies or work?

The most effective motivators are internal. Sure, you want to look your best, but if pleasing the eye is your only motivation, it's going to be pretty difficult to really develop healthy habits and find lasting weight loss.

In his book "Millionaire Success Habits," Dean Graziosi introduces the "seven levels deep" exercise. First, you write something you want. For example, "I want to lose weight." You then ask yourself "why" seven times, until you've reached a deep internal motivator.

Example: I want to lose weight

1. I want to lose weight because I want to be healthier.

2. I want to be healthier because I want to have more energy and stamina.

3. I want to have more energy so I can spend more quality time with my children.

4. I want to spend more time with my children, so they feel my love.

5. I want my children to feel my love, so they grow strong and healthy.

6. I want them to grow strong and healthy because they are important to me.

7. They are important to me because I love them.

As you can see, number seven, "because I love my children," is a very powerful motivator. You can remind yourself that you want to lose weight for your kids, not just for yourself.

Again, today's challenge is simply to consider and record your internal motivation. Try the seven levels deep exercise, then post it somewhere you can regularly review it.

Need additional support and motivation? Join our Facebook group! This is a community of people like you, with the purpose of supporting and motivating one another on our journeys to better health. Post any questions you have regarding health, and I will do my best to answer them in a timely manner. Or someone else in the group may respond to your post! Once there are 50 or more members in the group, I will start hosting live videos through the group. In each video I will address a different health topic and leave it open to questions at the end. This is a great opportunity for you to learn a little more about your health and get your questions answered. As detailed at the beginning of the book, this advice and any future advice I offer is not designed to replace the medical advice of a licensed professional. However, I only share information that is scientifically relevant and may assist you on your journey to better health. Scan the code to join:

Notes:

_____

_____

_____

_____

_____

_____

Day 12: Please, Don't Keto!

Pregnancy takes your body through some dramatic changes, including an increase in weight and fat storage. Even after your baby is born, excess fat in your body may be used to supply calories to your infant through breast milk. However, not everyone is able to breastfeed, and even women who do breastfeed may struggle to return to their pre-pregnancy weight.

Just to be clear, I hope that you recognize how incredible your body is! It was able to make the necessary changes to bring a new little life into the world. Gaining weight during that process is normal, as is a different body shape following pregnancy. This is something to be grateful for!

However, I know it can be hard for some to maintain a healthy weight following pregnancy, which is why we are discussing healthy ways to care for your body. It may be tempting to start an extreme diet plan to rapidly reduce your weight, but beware. As I am about to explain, even if a diet helps you lose weight, it may not be healthy in the long run.

You've likely heard of the keto diet, and the wild success stories of people following it. But what is it, and how does it work?

The keto diet relies on severely limiting carbs and replacing them with fats and proteins in your diet. Normally, when you eat a meal, carbs are converted into sugar and enter your bloodstream. This triggers the release of insulin. Insulin causes sugar to leave the bloodstream and enter your body cells. It also triggers fat storage. While this is a normal and healthy process, if you consume too much sugar at once, the sudden spike in blood sugar and insulin is not good for you. It's like slamming on the brakes. It safely stops your car but wears on the brakes and tires. Spikes in blood sugar increase fat storage within your body, and you quickly experience a sugar "crash," characterized by fatigue and hunger.

While it's a good idea to balance your meals to limit such spikes, the keto diet encourages cutting out almost all carbs. No carbs means no spikes in blood sugar, and very limited fat storage, fatigue, and hunger.

I knew someone who tried the keto diet for several weeks and almost completely cut carbohydrates out of his diet. I watched as his weight fell away, seemingly effortlessly. He didn't have to count calories or limit his food intake, just avoid carbs. Easy, right?

Of course, because the diet produced real results, he kept it up until one day he was forced to start incorporating carbs into his diet again, due to "undesirable side-effects." I tried to warn him!

While he didn't give me the specifics of these "undesirable side-effects," I can only guess what they might have been. When you cut carbs out of your diet, you are missing out on some pretty important nutrients.

Some important sources of carbs include whole grains, fruits and vegetables, nuts, and beans. These foods are high in fibers and lots of vitamins and minerals you cannot get from meat and fat sources alone. Fiber, for one, limits constipation and keeps your heart healthy. You do not want to miss out on this important nutrient!

While the keto diet may be great for weight loss, it's not necessarily great for your health in general. Interestingly, the keto diet was not originally designed for weight loss at all. It was recommended for patients experiencing brain dysfunctions such as seizures.

In addition, many keto dieters recommend eating lots of meats such as beef, pork, hot dogs, and sausages, which are high in saturated fats and not great for your overall health.

If you choose to follow the keto diet, make sure to include berries and vegetables, and consider taking a dietary supplement. As with any diet, it is super important to do your research before starting. Learn how to follow the diet in the safest way possible, what side effects may occur, and why the diet is effective.

What's your challenge for today? Pay attention to the carbs you eat. Write them down. At the end of the day, circle healthy sources of carbs and cross out the poor ones. Set a goal to fill your diet with more nutrient and fiber-dense sources of carbohydrates!

Nutrient and fiber-dense sources: berries (strawberries, raspberries, blueberries, blackberries), whole grains (whole wheat, oats, brown rice, quinoa), flax seed, chia seeds, nuts and seeds.

Poor sources: candy, sweets, baked goods, table sugar, white bread, white rice, starchy vegetables (potatoes, corn).

Notes:

_____

_____

_____

Day 13: Protein Bites Snack Recipe

I love protein bites, and they were an absolute lifesaver after the birth of my first baby. I had such a hard time finding a spare moment to eat or prepare food, so I relied heavily on snacks to keep my stomach relatively full. These protein bites were pretty quick and easy to make, so I would prepare a bunch at a time and keep them in the fridge. Whenever I got hungry, I could simply grab one of these healthy snacks, even while holding my baby. Packed with protein, omega-3 fatty acids, and dietary fiber, it was the perfect snack to keep me full and satisfied for longer than a few minutes.

You can find quite a variety of protein bite recipes on the internet with unique ingredients such as pumpkin, blueberry, and lemon. Some recipes require the use of protein powders. Make sure to scan the ingredients list and nutrition facts before purchasing any protein powder. Some powders contain a lot of added sugar, which isn't going to do you much good in the long run.

Peanut Butter Chocolate Protein Bites (makes 10 balls)

Ingredients:

4 dates
¼ cup water
½ cup peanut butter powder
¼ cup peanut butter
¾ cup oats
2 tbsp chia seeds or ground flaxseeds
¼ cup cocoa powder
¼ cup dark chocolate, chopped

Directions:

Blend dates and water in a blender on high until relatively smooth, about 20 seconds. Pour into a mixing bowl and add remaining ingredients. Stir until well combined, then roll into balls roughly 1-inch in diameter. Store in the refrigerator.

Notes:

_____

_____

_____

_____

_____

Peanut Butter Chocolate Protein Bites

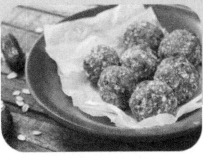

Serving size: 10 balls
Calories: 124

Prep time: 10 min
Cooking time: N/A

Ingredients

4 dates
¼ cup water
½ cup peanut butter powder
¼ cup peanut butter
¾ cup oats
2 tbsp chia seeds or ground flax seeds
¼ cup cocoa powder
¼ cup dark chocolate
chopped

Directions

1. Blend dates and water in a blender on high until relatively smooth, about 20 seconds.

2. Pour into mixing bowl and add remaining ingredients. Stir until well combined, then roll into balls roughly 1 inch in diameter. Store in refrigerator.

5g

4g

18g

4g

6g

Day 14: HIIT Workout

Daily affirmation: I am excited to wake up in the morning and live another day! I can't wait to see how the day unfolds!

HIIT stands for "high intensity interval training." As stated previously, HIIT workouts are great for boosting your metabolism, so you continue to burn fat throughout the day, even while resting. These exercises involve short, challenging bursts of activity, followed by active rest. Again, find a timer you can set up in front of you to keep track of each interval.

You may modify as needed: add weights or repeat exercises to increase intensity or perform smaller movements to decrease intensity. For example, jumping squats are quite intense, especially if you haven't worked out in a while. To reduce intensity, simply do regular squats, without the jump. Or for mountain climbers, you can hold the same position on the ground while stepping forward and backward, rather than jumping your feet alternately forward and backward.

Warm up:

30 sec arm circles forward

30 sec arm circles backward

30 sec jog in place

15 sec stand with legs wide apart and slowly reach down to touch the ground

15 sec reach over to right leg

15 sec reach over to left leg

Workout (repeat 3x):

45 sec high knees **(1)**

    20 sec walk in place

45 sec jumping squats **(2)**

    20 sec walk in place

45 sec mountain climbers **(3)**

    20 sec walk in place

45 sec jumping jacks

    20 sec walk in place

Cool down and stretch:

45 sec walk in place

15 sec stand on left foot. Lift right foot and grab with right hand. Pull foot gently towards your body to stretch front of thigh.

15 sec stand on right foot. Lift left foot and grab with left hand. Pull foot gently towards your body to stretch front of thigh.

10 sec stretch right arm across your chest

10 sec stretch right arm behind your back

10 sec stretch left arm across your chest

10 sec stretch left arm behind your back

Sit down with legs spread wide

15 sec reach towards your right foot

15 sec reach towards your left foot

Pull legs together, straight out in front of you

15 sec reach for your toes and pull them towards you for a calf stretch

Notes:

_____

_____

_____

_____

_____

_____

_____

_____

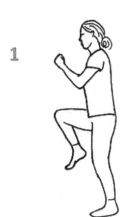

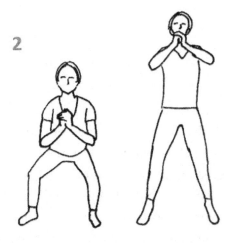

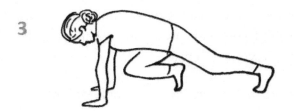

Day 15: Mid-Month Meditation

Daily affirmation: I am calm and peaceful.

Meditation is a great way to calm the mind and refocus on our priorities. We can let go of the little things that do not serve us and remind ourselves that we are safe, capable, and positive. Paired with progressive relaxation, meditation calms both mind and body, reducing the levels of stress hormones coursing through the blood. It helps us think more clearly, focus on what's most important, and make peaceful decisions. As you meditate, you quiet your mind. Your thoughts begin to heal and simplify.

Find a quiet place where you can focus on your breathing. If now is not a good time, wait until your kids are taking a nap, you get a break from work, or right before you go to bed.

Close your eyes and simply breathe. Take note of how you feel and how your body is moving. Focus on your body first: where do you feel relaxed? Where do you feel tense? Focus on your face, your shoulders, your core, etc. How is your stance? Is your back straight or rounded? How does your stomach feel? Are you hungry? Very full? Do you feel content? Now, focus on your mind: what thoughts are stepping onto the stage of your mind right now? What feelings come with those thoughts? What are you telling yourself? How do you feel as a mom? Anxious? Overwhelmed? Enthusiastic?

You are allowing yourself to feel and be just as you are. No need to change anything, just note where you are. Accept where you are without judgement or fear. Becoming aware of where you are now allows you to accept your mind and body in preparation to make gentle changes.

Sit or stand comfortably with your back straight and shoulders relaxed. Take a deep breath and squeeze your shoulders up to your ears. Clench your fists and the muscles in your face. As you exhale, roll your shoulders down and back, relax your hands and let them gently rest in your lap. Relax all the muscles in your face. Draw your attention to your feet. Relax all the muscles in your toes, and your feet, and then your ankles. Slowly work your way up your body until you feel all your muscles relax.

Continue your meditation by taking four deep breaths. Close your eyes, place one hand on your abdomen and one on your chest. As you breathe in, focus on expanding your abdomen rather than your chest.

Breathe in for one — two — three — four

Breathe out for one — two — three — four — five — six

Breathe in for one — two — three — four

Breathe out for one — two — three — four — five — six

As you breathe in, imagine you are drawing clean, fresh air into your lungs. You are filling your body with positivity and energy. As you breathe out, you are letting go of anything that is worrying you or causing you stress.

Breathe in for one — two — three — four — clean, fresh air

Breathe out for one — two — three — four — five — six — let go of the day

Breathe in for one — two — three — four — positivity and energy fill your body

Breathe out for one — two — three — four — five — six — release any remaining tension in your body

As you continue to breathe deeply, notice the little things around you. How does the chair feel beneath your legs? Or the floor beneath your feet. What sounds do you hear? The sound of your breath? If you are outside, can you feel the movement of the air? Hear the rustling of the leaves or even the grass? Gently draw your attention to the moment, letting go of any outside thoughts. Focus on your breathing. Don't worry about what you need to do today or tomorrow. Right now is just for you. Breathe, and relax.

Breathe in for one — two — three — four

Breathe out for one — two — three — four — five — six

Continue to breathe and repeat these phrases in your mind.

Anxiety does not serve me. It has no place in my life. Shame does not serve me. Let it go. Replace it with patience. I am capable. I am strong. I am confident. I am patient with myself and my shortcomings. I am learning a little each day. I am striving to reach my goals. I am mindful of where I am at right now. I am a wonderful mother. I make daily sacrifices to care for my baby. I accept my feelings without judgement. I am grateful for my emotions, because they alert me to the needs of my body. They help me take better care of myself. I can, and I will continue to grow more in-tune to the needs of my body.

At the end of your meditation, feel free to sit or lie down for a little longer and simply enjoy the stillness and simplicity of your thoughts.

Notes:

Day 16: Healthy Snacks

Daily affirmation: I live to give freely. I have an abundance to share with others.

Having snacks between meals can help keep your blood sugar level throughout the day. This means less hunger, more energy, and less unnecessary fat storage. But not just any snack will do the trick. So, what should you look for in your ideal snack?

Here are three qualities to keep in mind: protein, healthy fats, and fiber. These macronutrients slow digestion, keep you full longer, and reduce the effect of the meal on your blood sugar. For example, if you are looking for a good granola bar, check out the nutrition facts label before you buy. I like to have at least 5 grams of protein in my granola bars and 2 grams of fiber. I also look for bars with nuts which provide a great source of healthy fats and protein. In fact, many nuts and seeds are also good sources of fiber, which makes them perfect candidates for all three categories!

Certainly, while it's great to include at least one of these elements in your snack, it's even better if you can include all *three*. Strawberries are a great snack on their own (fiber source), but pair them with unsweetened

Greek Yogurt (protein source) and sliced almonds (protein and fat source), and you're golden!

Here's a list of some combo snacks you can include in your daily repertoire:

- Whole grain crackers, and celery with peanut butter
- Whole grain toast with peanut butter and banana slices
- Unsweetened Greek yogurt with granola, chopped walnuts, and blueberries
- Pistachios and raspberries
- Popcorn and roasted pecans
- Tuna mixed with a bit of mayonnaise on top of whole grain crackers or toast
- Hardboiled egg and avocado slices on top of whole grain toast

Today, in-between meals, pick two snack combos, or create your own. Your first snack should fall between breakfast and lunch, and your second snack between lunch and dinner. Make sure each snack has a protein, a fiber, and a healthy fat. If you are hungry before bed, you can have a snack then as well, but aim for foods very low in carbs.

If you do not yet have everything you need to make some healthy snacks today, make a grocery list! Stock up on foods from each of the three categories, so when it's snack time, you can easily grab what you need. A few examples have been listed below:

- Proteins: almonds, pistachios, pecans, peanuts, peanut butter, sunflower seeds, flax seeds, chia seeds, cheese, deli meat, chicken, turkey, tuna, eggs, yogurt (especially Greek yogurt), beans

- Fiber: flax seeds, chia seeds, strawberries, raspberries, blueberries, blackberries, whole grain bread and crackers, brown rice, oats, granola, beans

- Healthy fats: avocados, nuts, seeds, flax seeds, chia seeds, olive oil

Notes:

_____

_____

_____

_____

_____

_____

_____

_____

_____

_____

_____

Day 17: Protein, Fat, and Fiber

As stated earlier, protein, healthy fats, and fiber are three elements that slow digestion, keep you full longer, and promote energy. Every time you eat a meal or a snack, you should make sure at least one of these nutrients is included, ideally all three.

Protein can be divided into two categories: high-quality and low-quality. High-quality means the amino-acid profile closely matches that of the human body. In other words, you are getting the right ratios of building blocks your body needs to function. Low-quality proteins simply have a different profile of amino acids. They are not unhealthy by any means. You simply need to pair them with other low-quality proteins to supply your body with the correct ratio.

High-quality proteins come from animal products. Meats such as beef, chicken, and fish, as well as eggs and dairy products fall into this category. Many studies have shown that fish and poultry are the best meats for hearth health. However, red meats tend to be higher in iron, and occasionally enjoying a juicy steak isn't going to ruin your health.

Low-quality proteins include legumes (beans, peanuts), grains, nuts and seeds, and other plant foods. In order to supply the amino-acids, or protein building blocks, your body needs, you must eat both legumes and grains. This is especially important for vegetarians and vegans. If you eat meat on a regular basis, you are getting plenty of the right proteins and don't need to pair legumes and grains.

Now, what about fat? There are three types of fats we will discuss: trans, saturated, and unsaturated fats. Trans fats are the least healthy of the three and should be avoided at all costs. They've been strongly linked to heart disease, and because of this, are no longer found in many of the products you purchase from the grocery store. Saturated fats are found in animal products and are solid at room temperature. Besides the obvious streaks of fat found in meat products, this fat is also found in butter, cheese, and coconut oil. Generally, saturated fats are not great for your heart health.

The healthiest type of fat is unsaturated fat. Unsaturated fats come from plant sources and are liquid at room temperature. Examples include avocado oil, peanut oil, vegetable and canola oil, safflower oil, and olive oil. Some oils are rich in an even more specific type of fat called Omega-3 fatty acids, which are great for heart health and reducing inflammation. Foods rich in omega-3 fatty acids include flax seeds, chia seeds, and fish (especially salmon and other cold-water fish).

Fiber can also be divided into two sub-categories: soluble and insoluble. Soluble fiber is great for heart health and slows digestion, thus keeping you full longer. Insoluble fiber adds bulk to the stool and acts as a sort of scrub brush for the intestines, helping waste move on and out. Foods rich in fiber include nuts and seeds, fruits (especially berries like blueberries, blackberries, and raspberries), vegetables, whole grains, and legumes such as black beans and lentils.

Yesterday, you were challenged to include protein, fat, and fiber in your snacks, or at least make a grocery list to gather foods from each group.

Today, you will make sure your meals (breakfast, lunch, and dinner) have these three elements, plus a vegetable of your choice. You can write down what you plan to eat ahead of time, or when the meal arrives, consider what you have and eat something from each category. It may be helpful at first to print out a list of foods high in proteins, fats, and fibers and tape it to your fridge. That way you can easily reference what options you have and make an easy decision. Here are a few well-balanced meal suggestions to get you started:

- Turkey with whole-grain rolls and a salad with an olive-oil apple cider vinaigrette
- Chicken and red bell peppers (sauteed in olive oil) served with brown rice
- Burrito bowls with brown rice, beans, tomatoes, shredded lettuce, cilantro, grilled chicken, and sliced olives
- Deli meat sandwich on whole grain bread with mayonnaise, tomatoes, onions, and lettuce

Notes:

_____

_____

_____

_____

_____

_____

Day 18: Yoga Day!

Daily affirmation: I am calm and peaceful. My heart is at peace.

At a glance, you wouldn't think yoga was terribly impactful on your health. At least, *I* wouldn't. But the funny thing is that, towards the end of college, I actually started losing a significant amount of weight, and I gave a lot of the credit to my yoga workouts. Why?

The summer before my last couple of semesters, I was a lot more relaxed than usual. I wasn't taking classes, I was home with my family, I wasn't stressed about working or getting good grades, and I was finding peace with my body. Up until that point, I worried a lot about how I looked. I thought I was a little too round, my hair was too frizzy, my face was too greasy and scarred, and my acne wouldn't clear up all the way. But slowly, I started to accept my body and gain more confidence. My appreciation and gratitude for my health and my life increased.

During college, I was inconsistent with exercise but generally leaned towards higher-intensity workouts, anything that might maintain my weight or burn some of it away. But as I said, I really didn't lose weight until right before my final year, when I was no longer doing these heavy exercises. I was doing yoga, perhaps four or five times a week. I found all sorts of yoga videos on YouTube. Several of the instructors focused on drawing your attention to your body. I learned to focus on how I felt and how my body moved. I felt grateful for each movement, and when a pose was a little difficult, I welcomed the challenge and the burn in my muscles, because I knew my body loved the effort.

And the weight literally melted away. Effortlessly. Because I was not at all focused on trying to lose weight.

Stress plays a HUGE role in our overall well-being. I cannot emphasize this enough. I would argue that stress is one of the number one factors affecting our health. This villain seeps into our lives in the form of work, family responsibilities, school, relationships, past experiences, trauma, etc.

Even when you cannot rid yourself of the responsibilities and time constraints that fill your day, you *can* control your body's reaction to them. Your body physically responds to stress by releasing a hormone called cortisol. Ever heard of the fight or flight response? Cortisol is useful when you need to run from a bear or throw a burning car off your next-door neighbor, but it doesn't serve you well in day-to-day activities. Consistently high levels of cortisol increase hunger and weight gain, and the stress in general makes it harder to slow down and develop healthy habits.

So here are a few strategies you can use to limit your body's stress response and approach your day calmly and peacefully. First, take a deep breath. Breathing calmly and deeply several times in a row is a great way to reverse the stress response coursing through your veins. Place a hand on your abdomen as you breathe and focus on pushing that hand outward.

Second, take a five-minute break. I know, when you're in the middle of an important project, or even trying to break up a fight between your six-year-old and her older brother, it's hard to stop and take a break! But stepping out for just a moment to collect yourself, take a few deep breaths, walk around, stretch, or lay out on the lawn, can do wonders for your mental health. When you return, you will feel more calm, refreshed, and ready to tackle the task at hand.

Third, do yoga!

Now, I'm not a yoga instructor, and the yoga exercises I'm familiar with are very difficult to describe on paper. So today your challenge is to find a yoga video on YouTube and complete it. There is a wonderful variety of workouts to choose from: yoga for stress, yoga for weight loss, yoga for body image, power yoga, etc. You can choose a five-minute flow, or one that lasts an hour. It's up to you. If you don't have access to a yoga mat, your carpet will work just fine. Ready, set, relax!

Notes:

_____

_____

_____

_____

_____

_____

_____

_____

Day 19: A Breakfast for Champs

Daily affirmation: I wake up energized each morning. Drinking a full glass of water and eating a nutritious breakfast fuels my mind and body.

Remember learning about protein, fat, and fiber? Now, consider what you normally eat for breakfast and ask yourself, how does it measure against these nutrients? I'll be the first to admit that I LOVE breakfast cereal, and sadly it doesn't always measure high in protein, fat, and fiber. Unless I'm eating protein-fortified granola, I have a hard time finding cereal that meets such requirements without offending my taste buds. Though they are often fortified with lots of vitamins and minerals, great-tasting cereals tend to be high in sugar and rather low in protein, fats, and fibers. Generally, I like to add a scoop of peanut butter powder to the almond milk in my bowl to add a little boost of protein and fat.

But one of my favorite breakfasts to make is really very simple and easy, and very balanced. All you need is two frying pans, 5-10 minutes, and this recipe. I call them breakfast tacos, since they're eaten in a corn tortilla, but you can also use a whole-grain flour tortilla and wrap up the ingredients like a breakfast burrito. The corn tortillas are your carb sources, the avocado provides omega-3 fatty acids, the eggs are a great source of protein, and the veggies provide micronutrients such as vitamins A and C, calcium, and iron.

Breakfast Tacos

Ingredients:

2 corn tortillas
2 eggs, whisked
½ avocado, sliced
¼ cup pico de gallo or salsa
Optional: olive oil, red bell pepper, chopped spinach
Salt and pepper, to taste

Directions:

1. Set two frying pans on your stovetop and turn the heat to medium. Spray first pan with cooking spray and add eggs. Cook, gently scraping the bottom of the pan with a spatula as the eggs solidify.

2. When the second pan is hot, heat each tortilla in the pan on each side until crispy golden spots start to appear.

3. Spoon eggs evenly into the tortillas and top with pico de gallo and sliced avocados. Sprinkle with salt and pepper.

Variation: Pour olive oil and red bell peppers into one of the pans and sauté until soft. Push peppers to one side of the pan and add eggs to the empty spot (first spray with cooking spray if not using a non-stick pan). Cook, gently scraping the bottom of the pan as the eggs solidify. Add spinach and stir together with the bell peppers and eggs. Spinach should wilt as it heats up.

Breakfast Tacos

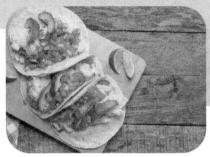

Serving size: 1
Calories: 330

Prep time: 5 min
Cooking time: 10 min

Ingredients

2 corn tortillas
2 eggs *whisked*
½ avocado *sliced*
¼ cup pico de gallo or salsa
Optional: olive oil, red bell pepper, chopped spinach
Salt and pepper *to taste*

Directions

1. Set two frying pans on your stovetop and set heat to medium. Cook eggs in first pan with cooking spray.

2. Heat corn tortillas in second pan until slightly crispy.

3. Spoon eggs, pico de gallo, and avocado slices into tortillas. Salt and pepper to taste.

15g
18g
29g
7g
2g

Notes:

_____

_____

_____

_____

_____

Day 20: Lower Body Ladders

Daily affirmation: My relationships with friends and family are fulfilling and joyful. We support each other as we make positive changes.

Ladder workouts are awesome for building muscle. They completely burn out the selected muscle group, leaving you shaky-legged and struggling to move. Not to mention the soreness the next day! Sounds great, right? But in all honesty, this is a pain I am happy to experience. I love the feeling of working hard and reaping the benefits. I feel energized, confident, and proud of my progress.

And the great news is that you won't experience such soreness every time you exercise. Each time you work out, your body's tolerance for lactic acid (which causes soreness) increases. It's totally worth it to push through the first few challenging exercises to reap the benefits of a leaner, meaner body!

Always remember to be proud of the efforts you take to improve your health! It's hard work, and you're rocking it!

But back to the ladder workouts. What exactly does that mean? A ladder exercise starts with a small number of repetitions with an equally long break, then gradually increases almost until you can't pump out any more repetitions. At that point, you start going back down the ladder. For example, you start with three squats, take a three second break, do four squats, take a four second break, and so on until you are doing ten squats followed by a ten second break. Then you start going back down. Nine squats with a nine second break, eight squats with an eight second break, all the way back down to three squats. You only need to do this once to completely wear out your muscles.

Today, you will be completing a lower body ladder workout. I will provide the list of exercises, and you will perform them in ladder format. Start by using the example format I just explained: three repetitions up to ten and back down to three. If you need to increase or decrease repetitions, you may do so.

Lower Body Ladder Workout

Squats: with feet shoulder-width apart and back straight, bend the knees to a 90-degree angle, then stand back up again. (1)

Side-lying leg-raises: lay on your right side with your right leg on the ground bent at an angle, and your left hand on the ground in front of you for support. Prop your head up on your right hand. Keep your top leg straight as you lift it up as high as you can without breaking form. Complete ladder exercise for this side, then repeat on the other side. (2)

Side-lying inner-leg raises: lay on your right side with your left leg straightened on the floor. Your top leg should be bent at a 90-degree angle with the foot resting on the ground in front of you. Your left hand should be on the ground in front of you for support, and your right elbow on the ground with your head resting on your hand. Lift the straight right leg away from the ground as high as you can. You will feel the burn in your inner thigh. Complete ladder exercise for this side, then repeat on the other side. (3)

Romanian deadlifts: stand on your left leg. Keep your right leg and back straight and in alignment as you reach down to touch the floor with your left hand. For greater resistance, put a weight in your left hand. The challenge of maintaining balance is what makes this such a great exercise, but if you really can't complete a repetition without falling over, keep a chair to your right and lightly hold it with your right hand. Complete ladder exercise on this side, then repeat on the next. You can also complete this exercise with both feet on the ground if this makes you more comfortable. (4)

Notes:

_____

_____

_____

_____

_____

_____

_____

_____

_____

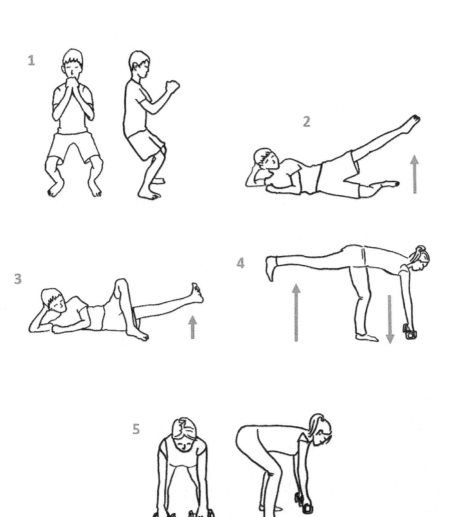

Day 21: Make Mistakes, and Make Them Often

Daily affirmation: I have unique strengths. I contribute positively to my family and community.

I would love to get better at public speaking. I've heard from several sources that a great way to improve your public speaking skills is by videotaping yourself speaking. You then watch the video, critique yourself, and try again. It's even more helpful if you write down what you did well and what you'd like to improve.

Sounds like a lot of work, though, doesn't it?

And the answer is yes. It is work. But the thing I fear most about beginning this exercise is not getting it right the first time.

Isn't that funny? The whole purpose of practicing is to get better and better each time. But often, when we try something new, we become discouraged when we don't quickly experience perfection. We are frustrated when we fall or mess up or fail to reap the benefits. Believe me, I am a HUGE culprit of this pattern of thinking.

But you know what? EVERY SINGLE TIME I have persistently practiced, something amazing has happened. I've *gotten better.* What? That's crazy, right?

The moral of the story is, please, please, please don't be afraid of failure. Don't be afraid of getting it wrong over, and over, and over, and over, and over again. Don't be afraid of starting a good thing in your life and perhaps giving up every now and then, or falling back into old habits, or not seeing results as quickly as you'd like to.

The reality is that you WILL fail every now and then, and that's okay! In fact, I would say it's a good thing to fail. Each time you make a mistake, you learn something from it. You haven't regressed. You've actually taken an important step forward!

And the more you fear failure, the less likely you will be to try in the first place. My mom always told me to be "gentle" with myself, and for good reason. She knew my tendency to get frustrated with failure and wanted me to succeed. She knew that every time I was willing to accept failure, I saw much more success.

When you mess up, when you spend a whole week doing nothing but watching TV, when you eat a whole bowl of ice cream even though you swore it off, when you start falling back into negative thought patterns, *be gentle with yourself.* You are, after all, human. And beating yourself up will only make the cycle worse. Accept the setback. Learn from it. Remind yourself that you are worthy, and capable, and awesome, and *human.* Then start over. Get back up and keep moving forward. It's going to be okay. I promise!

It's also important to focus on your strengths rather than focusing on your weaknesses all the time. There are definitely things you are good at, so what are they? Are you great at communicating? Connecting with people? Cooking? Organizing? Cleaning? Working? Whatever your strengths are, write them down. That is your challenge for today. Consider how you might use these strengths to aid you in your journey to better health. For example, if you're great at connecting with people, then reach out to a friend or group of friends to join you in each of these challenges! The mutual support will greatly increase your motivation and capacity for change.

Notes:

_____

_____

_____

_____

_____

_____

_____

_____

_____

_____

_____

_____

Day 22: Water

Daily affirmation: I feel so refreshed and full of life when I am well hydrated! I love the feeling of drinking cool, fresh water!

Imagine you're in the middle of a desert. The sun's hot, dry rays are beating down on you as you trek mindlessly towards the nearest source of water. The hot sand sifts through your sandals and toasts your toes. Sweat drips down the sides of your face and soaks the collar of your shirt. You blink rapidly to keep your eyes moist, but the effort is hardly doing the trick.

Thirsty yet?

Now imagine that after several miles of walking, you hear the faintest sound of rushing water. Could it be real? You pick up the pace in anticipation, running towards that beautiful noise. Finally, you step into a beautiful garden, your toes soothed by the cool, lush green grass. A glimmering waterfall splashes down into a bubbling brook that winds its way through bright flowers and sturdy shade trees. You rush forward and cup your hands under the ice-cold water and bring it to your lips, feeling the liquid cascade down your throat and fill you with renewed energy.

It's a pretty picture, isn't it?

I want you to imagine that your body is that beautiful garden. It is kept alive and thriving by a consistent source of clear water.

You're probably already aware that drinking water is important for your health. But why is it?

There are several reasons: your metabolism requires water to function properly. Your body is also made mostly of water. While you can go several days without food, your body will shut down much quicker without water. Drinking plenty of water keeps you energized and ensures that all systems are running at optimum capacity. Staying well hydrated also reduces your appetite and caloric intake, especially if you are replacing sweetened beverages (such as juice and soda) with water. Drinking a full glass of water before a meal can help trigger stretch receptors in the stomach that make you feel full, further reducing caloric intake.

How much water should you drink? One way to find out is to record your weight in pounds and divide it by two. That's how much you should be drinking in ounces. For example, if you weight 160 lbs, you need to drink 80 oz of water daily. To keep track, find a water bottle that holds a certain amount of water and calculate accordingly. If you need 80 oz of water each day, you could find a 32 oz water bottle and fill it up roughly three times. Or you can decide when to drink your water. You may drink a glass in the morning when you wake up, in between meals, and a couple hours before you go to bed.

Today, I want you to calculate your daily water needs, make a plan to meet them, then drink that much water throughout the day. I don't expect you to keep this every day from now on (though, if you do, that's great!). But I *do* want you to get a feel for how much water you should ideally be drinking every day. So today, drink the full amount. Then for the next few weeks, slowly increase the amount of water you drink each day until you are back up to the full amount you should be drinking. You can start with one water bottle for a week. Then the next week try filling up your water bottle twice. If you're used to drinking a lot of sugary beverages (like juice and soda) throughout the day, you may find that you drink less and less of them as your water intake increases.

Notes:

_____

_____

_____

_____

_____

_____

_____

_____

_____

_____

_____

_____

_____

Day 23: Salad Recipe

Daily affirmation: I am successful. I have no limits. I am excited to make positive changes and stick with them for the rest of my life.

I'll admit, I don't love eating salads, especially when I have to make them myself. The more ingredients and parts that go into a meal, the more overwhelming it feels. Often the only way I can prepare a full salad is by strapping my little girl into the baby carrier so she can come along for the ride. She doesn't like to miss out on the fun!

And for some reason, a salad tastes much better when assembled by someone else. However, with the right ingredients, a salad can be quite satisfying, and is certainly nutrient-packed. Here is one of my favorite salad recipes that can be eaten as a meal, not just on the side. It's packed with flavor, protein, fiber, unsaturated fats, and vitamins and minerals.

Meal prep tip: Try cooking all the chicken you will need for the week at once. Place several chicken breasts into an Instapot with two cups of water for 25 minutes (high pressure setting, rapid release). Or, cook in a crockpot on high for 4-6 hours or until chicken shreds easily with a fork. Cool, shred, and store chicken in the refrigerator to add to any recipe during the week!

Strawberry Balsamic Chicken Salad

Ingredients:

1 tbsp olive oil
1 clove garlic
1 chicken breast, sliced into thin strips
Salt and pepper
½ cup strawberries, halved
¼ cup almond slices
4 cups spinach
3 tbsp olive oil
3 tbsp balsamic vinegar
1 tsp honey
1 tsp Dijon mustard
Dash of salt and pepper
Optional: spring mix, cucumbers

Directions:

1. Heat olive oil in a frying pan over medium heat. Mince garlic and toss into the pan along with the chicken strips. Sprinkle salt and pepper on top. Sauté for roughly three minutes on each side, or until strips are golden brown and cooked through.

2. For the dressing, combine olive oil, balsamic vinegar, honey, Dijon mustard, salt and pepper in a blender for about ten seconds. Toss dressing with spinach, strawberries, almond slices, and chicken. You can also add in spring mix and sliced cucumbers for a little more variety.

Strawberry Balsamic Chicken Salad

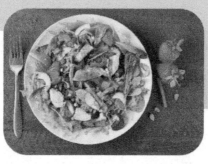

Serving size: 4
Calories: 316

Prep time: 10 min
Cooking time: 10 min

Ingredients

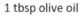

1 tbsp olive oil
1 clove garlic
1 chicken breast *sliced*
Salt and pepper
½ cup strawberries *halved*
¼ cup almond slices
4 cups spinach
Optional: spring mix, cucumbers

Dressing
3 tbsp olive oil
3 tbsp balsamic vinegar
1 tsp honey
1 tsp Dijon mustard
Dash of salt and pepper

Directions

1. Sauté garlic and chicken strips in hot olive oil in a frying pan over medium heat. Sprinkle with salt and pepper.

2. Combine dressing ingredients in a blender until smooth. Toss with remaining salad ingredients.

15g
25g
9g
2g
5g

Notes:

_____

_____

_____

_____

_____

Day 24: Sleep for You and Your Baby

Daily affirmation: My feelings are valid. I accept them without judgement and allow them to run their course. I seek safe and healthy ways to care for these emotions.

As you are well aware, sleep is one of the hardest things to tackle following childbirth. In the beginning, your little one needs to be fed every couple of hours both day and night, so you never get to sleep for long. If you're like me, it probably takes you a while to fall asleep in the first place, so you're just barely settling into a restful sleep when it's time to feed again!

After the first few weeks, your baby may start sleeping for longer stretches at night. Around four months, it may get worse again as your baby's sleep patterns mature. He starts to wake more fully after each sleep cycle, which means it's harder for him to fall back asleep on his own. You may begin to consider sleep training within the next couple of months (see "Sleep training" section in this chapter).

Sleep can impact your health on many different levels. For one, when you cut your sleep short, the part of your brain designed to regulate

101

emotions doesn't function properly. Your stress levels go up. You may be more irritable or anxious; and as we discussed previously, more stress means more cortisol, which isn't great for your health.

Sleep also helps regulate your metabolism, your appetite, and your ability to make good choices. Have you ever noticed that when you stay up late or don't sleep enough, that you get hungry? And I'm willing to bet the first thing you go for to satisfy that hunger isn't a salad.

Personally, I find the quantity of sleep a little harder to tackle than the quality of sleep, due to all the external factors demanding your time. This is certainly a challenge when you have a newborn. When my baby was born, I was counseled to do everything I could to get enough sleep. That meant accepting a LOT of help from family and friends. I didn't love it, because I was *sure* I could push through each day enough to make dinner, keep the house clean, and care for my baby on what little sleep I was getting. I didn't want to nap during the day when my baby was napping, because it gave me time to finally get stuff done. But it wasn't long before my body crashed and I *had* to sleep, or I simply could not function, emotionally or physically. I *had* to accept the fact that not everything was going to get done each day, and I tried to welcome what help was offered.

Consider what you might be able to adjust in your schedule to make sure you are getting your z's. Do you need to start getting ready for bed earlier? Put your phone down more frequently so you can get your work done a little sooner? Set timers? Sleep when baby is napping? Organize your daily schedule? Accept a little help from family or friends?

And of course, even if you are getting *enough* sleep, it won't do you much good if the *quality* of your sleep is poor. Your body goes through several sleep cycles throughout the night, switching from light sleep (or REM sleep) to deeper levels of sleep on repeat. Every part of this cycle is vital for your health, and if compromised, will affect your habits, emotions, and well-being during the day. REM sleep, for example, contributes to emotional health, stress, and memory.

In order to improve the quality of your sleep and make sure your cycles are complete and healthy, there are a few steps you can take.

1. Establish a bedtime routine. Brush your teeth, bathe, change your clothes, read for a few minutes, then turn out the light. It doesn't matter much *what* you do, so long as you do the same thing every night. Keeping a consistent bedtime routine signals to your body that it's time to start winding down for sleep.

2. Turn off the phone an hour and a half before going to bed. Staring at a screen right before going to bed can mess with your circadian rhythm since the light mimics the sunlight of day. In addition, the "blue light" emitted from screens has been shown to negatively impact sleep.

3. Start winding down a couple hours before bed. Avoid exercising, playing intense games, or working on anything that gets you really riled up. Believe me, this one can be hard! Oftentimes, the best time for me to work on passion projects is right before I go to bed, since the kids are sleeping, and the house is quiet. But I do sleep better when I allow my brain to slow down a bit before hitting the hay.

Today's challenge is to take five minutes to do a little research of your own. Type the words "sleep and health" (or "sleep and weight loss" if you are trying to lose weight) into your web browser, and pick an article to read. There's a lot of interesting information out there, and taking a little time to get informed can do wonders for your motivation. You may be surprised to note just how important your sleep is and what a great impact it has on your health! Write in your journal what you've learned and pick one thing you'd like to do to get more sleep, or to improve the quality of your sleep. Tonight, make sure you stick with your goal!

Sleep Training

Is your baby five months old or older? Do you rock your baby to sleep every night? Are you exhausted by the nighttime routine? Does your baby scream and cry excessively at bedtime? Are you ready to finally get eight hours of sleep?

Being at least five months old is crucial to the success of sleep training. While some babies learn to sleep through the night much earlier, it is not a good idea to intentionally "train" a baby so young. Infants do not know how to soothe themselves to sleep. If your infant cries herself to sleep before five months, her sleep is more likely due to exhaustion than skill. After five months, most babies are capable of soothing themselves.

We first sleep-trained at five months with my little girl. The first three nights were brutal, especially the third night. It went against every bone in my body to let her cry like that. Her crib was in our room, and we had a one-room apartment at the time. So, there was no way to separate myself from the cries to make it easier to bear.

But, on the fourth night, she miraculously slept through the whole night without waking. And then the next night was the same. When we laid her down in her crib at night, she would get comfortable and fall asleep on her own. It was such a relief!

Unfortunately, I was not consistent after that, and we fell back into some poor sleep habits. At seven months, we decided to sleep train again, but then she got sick. And then my husband got sick. And then my stepdaughter got sick. And then I got sick. And then our baby girl got sick again. And then I got sick again! It was such a mess!

But, luckily, after all the crazy, we managed to sleep train again, and I am happy to say that she is sleeping much better, and so are we. You don't realize how much sleep affects you until you lose it for several months and suddenly get it back!

My experience with sleep training was rough, to say the least. However, I continue to recommend it to friends and family because in the end, it worked! My baby started sleeping through the night without waking, which gave me a much better chance at rest.

There are several different sleep training methods out there. Some are advertised as the "no cry" method, which sounds appealing but, in my opinion, is a little deceptive. No mother wants to ignore her baby's cries. It is both heart-wrenching and biologically challenging. We, as mothers, simply weren't wired to let our babies cry! But if you decide to sleep train your baby, some level of tears is inevitable. Your baby loves being with you, and sleeping on his own is a difficult change to make!

Keep in mind that if your baby is already crying a lot during the nighttime routine, this isn't much different. You are simply giving that crying a purpose.

Steps to successfully sleep train your baby

Establish a nighttime routine: give her a bath, put on pajamas, feed her, read her a story, turn on the sound machine, and lay her in her crib awake. It doesn't matter much what you choose to do, as long as the routine is the same every night. This tells your baby it's time to start winding down.

Choose a bedtime between 7-8pm. Experts say this is the best time to put your baby to bed for a good night's sleep. If he is going to bed pretty late right now, slowly bring the time closer to 8pm each night until his body adjusts to the earlier bedtime.

Once baby is in bed, leave the room. Check in on her after five minutes, then ten minutes, then every fifteen minutes until she falls asleep. If she is starting to calm down at any of these intervals, do not go check on her (unless you need to for some reason). "Checking in" means rubbing her belly, smoothing her hair, speaking in a gentle whisper, etc. Don't pick her up or try to rock her to sleep.

Schedule feedings. If your baby is older than five months, she should be able to go the whole night without eating. However, it is different for all babies. We continued to maintain night feedings until our baby was seven months old before successfully weaning her. If you choose to continue feeding at night, schedule 1-2 feedings and do not deviate from these times. For example, you may schedule feedings for 11pm and 3am. If your baby wakes at any other time, you will let her cry back to sleep, checking in as you did at bedtime. Then, at the scheduled times, you will pick up your sleeping baby and feed her. Sometimes she will eat in her sleep, and other times she may be too deep in sleep to eat. If she does not eat, you may set her back down and try again in another half hour.

Always use your motherly intuition. If you believe something is wrong, don't hesitate to check in on your baby. Her safety is of utmost importance.

If you follow the steps consistently, your baby should be sleeping through the night by the end of two weeks. It may seem cruel, but the consistency tells your baby, "When you are in your crib, it is time to sleep." If you sometimes pick her up when she is crying, this confuses her.

You can go into much greater depth on sleep training here.

Notes:

Day 25: Upper Body Ladders

This is the one workout I'm giving you that requires some sort of weights for each exercise. However, if you don't own any, just grab a couple of water bottles, and they'll do just fine! Remember, this is an upper body *ladder* workout, so we will start with a small number of repetitions and gradually increase until we can't do much more. Then we will decrease back to where we started. If you are using lighter weights, or water bottles, or cans, and you reach the top of the ladder without much of a burn, simply extend your ladder. Continue to increase your repetitions until your arms are sore, then start to go back down the ladder. Ready? Here we go!

Exercise tip: Try exercising in the morning, at midday, and in the evening to find what time works best for you. Of course, it may change from day to day, because motherhood is so unpredictable! But if you consistently struggle to exercise at the end of the day when you're dead exhausted, try exercising during nap time or getting up a little early.

Warm up

Arm circles forward and backward for 15 seconds each. Stretch your arms across the front of your chest for 15 seconds on each side, then reach above and bend your elbow to touch your back. Gently press on your elbow and hold the stretch for 15 seconds on each side.

Gently rotate your torso to swing your arms from side to side for 20 seconds.

Workout

For each of these exercises, start with 5 repetitions, take a 5 second break, then do 6 repetitions with a 6 second break, until you reach 20 repetitions. Then work your way back down to 5 repetitions. If your muscles reach exhaustion before 20 repetitions, stop where you are at and work your way back down the ladder. Make sure to stretch after completing the workout.

Bicep curls (1)

Triceps extensions (2)

Shoulder presses (3)

Bent over rows: you may keep both legs together as you bend forward with a flat back, then do rows with both arms simultaneously. OR, you may step back with one leg, rest the opposite arm on the front bent leg, and do rows with the free arm (4) (see illustrations).

Lateral raises (5)

Bent over deltoid fly (6)

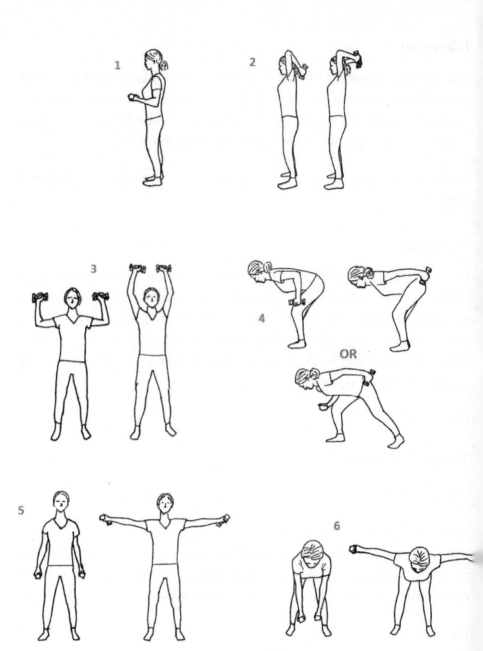

Notes:

Day 26: Keep a Food Diary

Did you know that the first sign of hunger is actually just thinking about food? Responding to hunger cues as quickly as possible is important to maintaining a healthy diet. By the time you get that empty feeling in your stomach, your ability to mindfully select a nutritious food is significantly impaired. One way to pay closer attention to these hunger cues is by keeping a food diary. Throughout the day, stop every couple of hours and take a minute to note how you are feeling. Write it down in a little notepad, or in a notes app on your phone. Set an alarm for every two hours if needed to remind you to pause.

Keeping a food diary is also a great way to figure out what foods suit you and what foods don't. For example, if you tend to get a lot of abdominal cramping but don't know what food is the cause, it's helpful to write down everything you eat throughout the day, and how you feel throughout the day. Eventually, you will start to recognize a pattern.

Perhaps when you drink milk, you notice the cramping two hours later. Now you know what you need to remove from your diet.

Record keeping is great for developing healthy lifestyle changes as well. It does require a little time and effort, but if you keep your notebook handy and just take a couple seconds to jot down information, it's really not much of a commitment. To complete your food diary today, grab a sheet of paper. You can also try searching "food diary" on the internet and will likely find some templates already created for you. But if you want to make a simple sheet of your own, take your paper and make two columns, making the right a little wider. On the left, you will write times. On the right, you will record what you eat (at meals), and how you feel. If you eat your breakfast at 8am, on the left column record the time 8am. On the right, record the eggs and toast you ate, and roughly how much (ex: 2 slices of toast, 2 fried eggs). Perhaps at 9:30am, you find yourself getting hungry. Again, record the time on the left, and on the right, write that you are getting hungry. Continue this pattern throughout the day, paying attention to your eating and snacking patterns, and how you feel before, after, and in-between meals. At the end of the day, assess your food diary. What patterns do you notice? Do you get hungry quicker after eating certain meals or snacks? Do you have any cramping? Excessive fullness?

Food diaries are most effective when kept over long periods of time. However, even this quick snapshot into your health habits can be eye-opening and increases your awareness.

Notes:

_____

_____

_____

_____

_____

_____

_____

_____

_____

_____

_____

_____

_____

_____

Day 27: Healthy Dessert Recipe

Daily affirmation: I am comfortable making mistakes. I love learning from the paths I take, both good and bad.

When I was in my junior year of high school, I decided I'd go a whole year without eating treats. This meant no ice cream, cookies, brownies, cake, candy, chocolate, etc. For the first few weeks, it was a little challenging, but after that, I really didn't crave the sugar at all. I quickly found other delicious foods I enjoyed, and the hardest part was simply not participating in the cultural celebrations we're all so used to. It's hard to attend a birthday party, wedding, movie night, or any other occasion without encountering sweets of some sort. However, if you are really committed to improving your diet, others will notice and eventually stop offering you junk food. They may even join the healthy habit train!

But for those days when you really want something sweet, or something to sit back and enjoy while you read a good book, here's one of my favorite dessert recipes. It's not sugar free, but all the sugars here come from relatively healthy sources like agave nectar and fruit. And if you need a vegan option, you can replace the cream cheese with vegan cream cheese, and it's still delicious!

No-Bake Cheesecake for One

Ingredients

2 tbsp cream cheese, vegan or regular, softened
1 tsp agave nectar
1 tsp lemon juice
¼ tsp vanilla extract
¼ tsp lemon zest
¼ cup coconut whipped cream
1 tbsp almond flour
1 tbsp coconut flour
1 tsp coconut oil
2 tbsp fresh raspberries

Directions

1. With a hand mixer, blend cream cheese, agave nectar, lemon juice, vanilla, and lemon zest for 2 minutes or until smooth. Fold in whipped cream.

2. Combine flours and oil and press into the bottom of a cupcake liner or small bowl. Spoon cheesecake filling on top. Chill and serve with raspberries.

No-bake Cheesecake for One

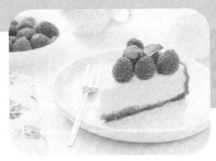

Serving size: 1
Calories: 266

Prep time: 10 min
Cooking time: N/A

Ingredients

2 tbsp cream cheese *vegan or regular, softened*
1 tsp agave nectar
1 tsp lemon juice
¼ tsp vanilla extract
¼ tsp lemon zest
¼ cup coconut whipped cream
1 tbsp almond flour
1 tbsp coconut flour
1 tsp coconut oil
2 tbsp fresh raspberries

Directions

1. With a hand mixer, blend cream cheese, agave nectar, lemon juice, vanilla, and lemon zest for 2 minutes or until smooth. Fold in whipped cream.

2. Combine flours and oil and press into the bottom of a cupcake liner or small bowl. Spoon cheesecake filling on top. Chill and serve with raspberries.

4g
21g
15g
5g
9g

Notes:

_____

_____

_____

_____

_____

Day 28: Not All Sugar is Created Equal

Did you know that sugars from different sources have a different impact on your blood sugar? The most basic sugar molecules in your diet are fructose, glucose, and galactose. Each of these sugars consists of a single sugar molecule, called a monosaccharide. Monosaccharides pair up to form the next level of sugar molecules, disaccharides. A fructose and a glucose molecule make sucrose, which is the sugar you normally use in baking. Two glucose molecules form maltose, and a glucose and a galactose molecule form lactose, the sugar found in milk. These monosaccharides and disaccharides are commonly referred to as "simple sugars," and are generally digested very quickly. Consequently, they tend to impact your blood sugar rather dramatically, especially when eaten alone.

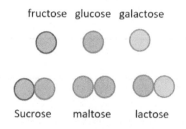

Complex carbohydrates, on the other hand, are made of long chains of glucose and generally digest more slowly than simple sugars. This means a slower and more beneficial effect on your blood sugar.

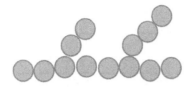

However, there are some exceptions to this rule, as identified by the glycemic index.

The glycemic index assigns numbers to different foods based on how quickly they cause your blood sugar to rise. The higher the number, the quicker the food is converted into simple sugars that enter your bloodstream.

White bread, for example, is higher on the glycemic index than table sugar. This means that white bread more quickly spikes your blood sugar. Even though bread consists of complex carbohydrates, white bread has been stripped of the healthy fats and fibers that normally slow digestion.

Here's your assignment for today. On the internet, find a glycemic index chart, print it out, review it, and tape it to your fridge. Look for a chart that covers foods you commonly eat. You may be surprised to find what foods place highest on the glycemic index! Remember, we generally want to avoid foods that rank high on the glycemic index. Lower numbers are better for your health and weight loss.

Notes:

_____

_____

_____

_____

_____

_____

_____

_____

_____

_____

_____

_____

_____

_____

Day 29: A Word on Mindless Eating

Daily affirmation: I have a loving support system and am capable of overcoming trial.

I think a lot of people have a hard time starting something because they are stressed about getting it right the first time. For example, it took me a long time to finally write and finish my first book because I wanted to publish a flawless and awe-inspiring book right off the bat. And this isn't uncommon among authors. Often, people wait to write a book because when they sit down to write, they want to have everything perfectly written and organized right away. And as life continues, they never find the perfect moment to start.

Become the best you. Don't worry about how many walks your neighbor takes, or what home-cooked meals your best friend is preparing. It's not a race or a competition. You cannot be compared with anyone else. Just become the best you. Strengthen your mind and body a little each day, and work towards realistic goals.

One last item to address is mindless eating. Have you ever sat down to watch your favorite television show with a huge bag of chips, only to discover in horror that the entire bag was empty within the hour? Certainly, you didn't plan to eat the whole bag by yourself! Why didn't your stomach warn you to stop?

Mindless eating is a huge issue because it dramatically reduces the number of senses triggered by a meal. Your brain takes in a lot of information from different parts of the body to know when you are full. In turn, it sends out signals to let your body know it's time to stop eating. The stomach, for one, has stretch receptors which trigger "fullness," or satiety when there is a lot of food in the stomach.

However, your overall eating experience plays a huge role in how satisfied you feel after a meal. Smelling, tasting, feeling, seeing, and even hearing your food contribute to satisfaction and satiety. This is why mindless eating can be such a problem. Eating while watching TV, scrolling through your phone, working on the computer, or even remembering a stressful conversation limits your awareness. Distractions divert your attention from a meal, making it difficult to notice when you really are full. And even when your stomach *feels* full, you may not *mentally* feel fully satisfied and may continue to eat.

It is important to separate eating from your other daily activities. Take time to establish a positive setting for mealtimes. Get the family involved. Sit around the table and enjoy one another's company while eating. Talk and allow yourselves to take your time enjoying the meal. This is one part of your day that should not be rushed.

If you do like to snack while watching movies or TV, consider portioning out your snack in advance. Pour your chips into a small bowl or baggie, put a handful of nuts into a napkin, spoon some veggie dip onto a plate aside your favorite vegetables, etc. This can prevent the whole, "Whoops! I just ate an entire bag of chips!" scenario.

Today's challenge is all about changing your mindset. Instead of seeing healthy eating as a chore, we want to enjoy and relish the nutrient packed foods we eat.

You are going to treat yourself to a nutritious meal and sit down to enjoy it. It doesn't have to be anything expensive or elaborate, just something healthy you can genuinely appreciate. Find veggies with lots of color to add to a salad. Try grilling some chicken with a new seasoning. Slice up some fruits to decorate your dinner plate.

Make sure the environment is free from distractions. As you eat, focus on your food and enjoy every bite. Express gratitude for the variety in color, taste, and texture in your meal. Take a moment to appreciate how good you feel after fueling your body with such nutritious foods.

As you progress along your fitness journey, you will learn to enjoy and love your new healthy habits. Consequently, the habits will stick. Embrace your newfound energy and strength. Treat yourself to delicious, nutritious meals and snacks and don't be afraid to experiment and get creative. Take your baby to the farmers market and find some fresh locally grown produce. Learn some fun simple food garnishes to dress up your meals. Enjoy the journey!

Notes:

_____

_____

_____

_____

_____

_____

Day 30: Conclusion

Daily affirmation: I am proud of myself for completing this challenge and excited to keep learning. Positive changes are a regular part of my life. I am a great mom!

Remember in the introduction, how we discussed the example of the mechanic? We know that every broken car requires a different fix, and the same goes for our bodies. Have you discovered yet what might be broken? Let's review the different techniques, strategies, and potential fixes that we've discussed over the past 30 days:

- Balancing proteins, fats, and carbohydrates (including fiber)
- Doing strength exercises to build muscle and boost your metabolism
- Relieving stress through yoga, meditation, and mindfulness
- Healthy snacking
- Getting adequate, good quality sleep

Which one(s) do you think you need to continue working on? Which one(s) would you like to delve into more? Take a look at the journal you've kept over the past month and consider which challenges made the biggest impact on your health.

My hope is that by applying these techniques, you will not only lose weight, but improve your overall health. I hope you find more energy, more peace, and greater motivation along your journey. And please, never stop learning. The more you read, the more you expose yourself to information regarding your health, the more likely you will be to apply these principles. The more likely you will be to take action and make healthier lifestyle changes. Supposedly the average person must be exposed to a particular advertisement seven times before deciding to make a purchase. And if our decisions to live healthier are at all similar, we ought to expose ourselves to whatever educational materials we can get our hands on.

Remember that the key to improving your health is making small, permanent lifestyle changes. Don't expect to perfect your health all at once. Hopefully, this will be a journey you take for the rest of your life. Don't be afraid to keep learning and trying new things. Just don't ever give up. Be persistent and willing to work hard. Your health is important. It affects every aspect of your life. Guard it. Take care of it, and it will take care of you.

So, what's your final challenge? Choose one of the techniques you've learned over the past month and dive a little deeper. Write down questions you have, do a little research, and apply what you learn. And keep repeating this until you've developed some solid, healthy habits in your life! Then, pass on what you've learned, or share along the way. Take your friends and family with you on your journey to greater health!

You got this, mama!

Notes:

_____

_____

_____

_____

_____

_____

_____

_____

_____

_____

_____

_____

_____

_____

_____

Bonus: For Working Moms

Daily affirmation: I am an awesome mom!

Whether you work from home or go out for your day job, you are busy, to say the least. It can be hard to find a balance between work and family responsibilities, and you frequently feel overwhelmed and tired. How are you supposed to find the time to exercise, feed your family, go to work and everything, and stay sane!

Be assured that you are not alone in your challenges. You will likely never find perfect "balance," and that is okay. Some days, you may have more work responsibilities. Others, you may spend time with your family. The sacrifices of love that you make for your family will be recognized, if not now, when your kids are grown. When they start families of their own, they will be grateful for your example and your care. I am certainly much more grateful for all my mom has done, now that I am a mom myself!

That being said, what are some strategies you can employ to improve work/life balance and make time for self-care?

Exercise daily. Find something you enjoy, and stick with it. I love going for walks because my baby is content, and I get some fresh air. It's a no-brainer to do this exercise daily! You may enjoy dancing, running, jogging, tennis, swimming, etc. Enjoying a little exercise each day will be excellent for both your physical and mental health. You will be able to think more clearly, and your productivity will improve.

Keep things separate. This is much more difficult if you work from home, as I do. My mind is almost constantly caught up with ideas and the never-ending list of things to do. Sometimes when I am with my kids, I am so distracted that it's hard to give them my full love and attention, which they need! I find it helpful to write my thoughts down in my phone so I can remove them from my mind. When I am with my kids or my spouse, I try to keep my phone at a distance.

Write things down. I mentioned this in the previous bullet. Keeping a written to-do list and recording your thoughts and ideas can reduce overwhelm. It's comforting to know that you have everything written down, so you won't forget it.

Take time for yourself. I know how hard it is to make time to do something you love, but it's important! When I got married, I was very overwhelmed by my new role as mother (to my stepdaughter). It was difficult to go from complete independence to caring for another little human. I would often wake up dreading the day ahead. It was a horrible feeling! But as soon as I picked up a passion project, I started to wake up each day full of excitement. It was rejuvenating to keep learning and working on something I loved.

Eat a balanced diet. Eating well strengthens your body and mind and makes daily tasks easier.

Keep a gratitude journal. Focusing on your challenges only makes them more challenging. At the end of the day, write one thing you are grateful for. You will start to see your life in a more positive light.

Notes:

_____

_____

_____

_____

_____

_____

_____

_____

_____

_____

_____

_____

_____

_____

_____

_____

Go ahead! Write it down! What's the first topic or health habit you'd like to develop a little further?

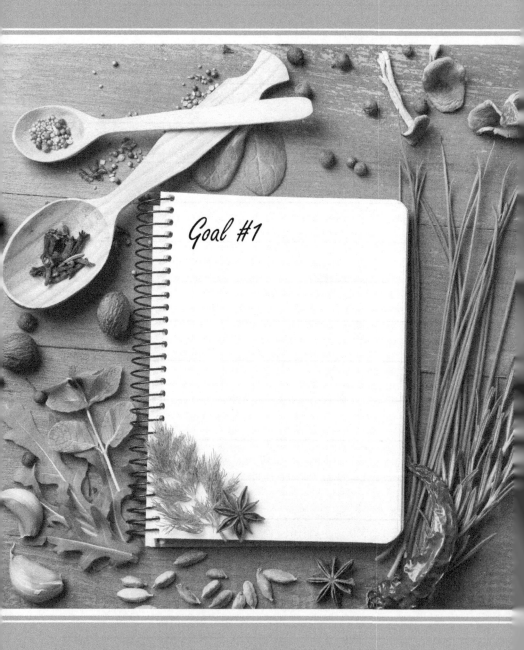

Goal #1

Today is the first day of the rest of your life!

References

1. Beware high levels of cortisol, the stress hormone. Feb 5, 2017. https://www.premierhealth.com/your-health/articles/women-wisdom-wellness-/beware-high-levels-of-cortisol-the-stress-hormone

2. Geary N. Control-theory models of body-weight regulation and body-weight-regulatory appetite. Appetite. 2020 Jan 1;144:104440. doi: 10.1016/j.appet.2019.104440. Epub 2019 Sep 5. PMID: 31494154.

3. Graziosi, D. (2019). Millionaire success habits: The gateway to wealth & prosperity. Hay House, Inc.

4. Kelly E. What you need to know about anaerobic exercise. Modified Mar 6, 2019. https://www.healthline.com/health/fitness-exercise/anaerobic-exercise.

5. Luat AF, Coyle L, Kamat D. The Ketogenic Diet: A Practical Guide for Pediatricians. Pediatr Ann. 2016 Dec 1;45(12):e446-e450. doi: 10.3928/19382359-20161109-01. PMID: 27975114.

6. Lyzwinski LN, Caffery L, Bambling M, Edirippulige S. The Mindfulness App Trial for Weight, Weight-Related Behaviors, and Stress in University Students: Randomized Controlled Trial. JMIR Mhealth Uhealth. 2019 Apr 10;7(4):e12210. doi: 10.2196/12210. PMID: 30969174; PMCID: PMC6479283.

7. Morris MJ, Beilharz JE, Maniam J, Reichelt AC, Westbrook RF. Why is obesity such a problem in the 21st century? The intersection of palatable food, cues and reward pathways, stress, and cognition. Neurosci Biobehav Rev. 2015 Nov;58:36-45. doi: 10.1016/j.neubiorev.2014.12.002. Epub 2014 Dec 10. PMID: 25496905.

8. Payne ME, Porter Starr KN, Orenduff M, Mulder HS, McDonald SR, Spira AP, Pieper CF, Bales CW. Quality of Life and Mental Health in Older Adults with Obesity and Frailty: Associations with a Weight Loss Intervention. J Nutr Health Aging. 2018;22(10):1259-1265. doi: 10.1007/s12603-018-1127-0. PMID: 30498835; PMCID: PMC6444357.

9. Schvey NA, Puhl RM, Brownell KD. The stress of stigma: exploring the effect of weight stigma on cortisol reactivity. Psychosom Med. 2014 Feb;76(2):156-62. doi: 10.1097/PSY.0000000000000031. Epub 2014 Jan 16. PMID: 24434951.

10. Shai I, Schwarzfuchs D, Henkin Y, Shahar DR, Witkow S, Greenberg I, Golan R, Fraser D, Bolotin A, Vardi H, Tangi-Rozental O, Zuk-Ramot R, Sarusi B, Brickner D, Schwartz Z, Sheiner E, Marko R, Katorza E, Thiery J, Fiedler GM, Blüher M, Stumvoll M, Stampfer MJ; Dietary Intervention Randomized Controlled Trial (DIRECT) Group. Weight loss with a low-carbohydrate, Mediterranean, or low-fat diet. N Engl J Med. 2008 Jul 17;359(3):229-41. doi: 10.1056/NEJMoa0708681. Erratum in: N Engl J Med. 2009 Dec 31;361(27):2681. PMID: 18635428.

11. Stookey JD, Constant F, Popkin BM, Gardner CD. Drinking water is associated with weight loss in overweight dieting women independent of diet and activity. Obesity (Silver Spring). 2008 Nov;16(11):2481-8. doi: 10.1038/oby.2008.409. Epub 2008 Sep 11. PMID: 18787524.

12. Tinsley G. 7 benefits of high-intensity interval training (HIIT). Modified Jun 2, 2017. https://www.healthline.com/nutrition/benefits-of-hiit.

13. Viana RB, Naves JPA, Coswig VS, de Lira CAB, Steele J, Fisher JP, Gentil P. Is interval training the magic bullet for fat loss? A systematic review and meta-analysis comparing moderate-intensity continuous training with high-intensity interval training (HIIT). Br J Sports Med. 2019 May;53(10):655-664. doi: 10.1136/bjsports-2018-099928. Epub 2019 Feb 14. PMID: 30765340.

14. Westcott WL. Resistance training is medicine: effects of strength training on health. Curr Sports Med Rep. 2012 Jul-Aug;11(4):209-16. doi: 10.1249/JSR.0b013e31825dabb8. PMID: 22777332.

15. Wewege M, van den Berg R, Ward RE, Keech A. The effects of high-intensity interval training vs. moderate-intensity continuous training on body composition in overweight and obese adults: a systematic review and meta-analysis. Obes Rev. 2017 Jun;18(6):635-646. doi: 10.1111/obr.12532. Epub 2017 Apr 11. PMID: 28401638.

16. Zhang H, Tong TK, Qiu W, Zhang X, Zhou S, Liu Y, He Y. Comparable Effects of High-Intensity Interval Training and Prolonged Continuous Exercise Training on Abdominal Visceral Fat Reduction in Obese Young Women. J Diabetes Res. 2017;2017:5071740. doi: 10.1155/2017/5071740. Epub 2017 Jan 1. PMID: 28116314; PMCID: PMC5237463.

Additional Readings

- "Power of Habit: Rewire Your Brain to Build Better Habits and Unlock Your Full Potential"

- "Happy Here and Now: Lasting Happiness You Can Count On," by Matt Tracy

- Check out my blog for more recipes and tips for new moms: www.onapenny.com/blog

- **Other books by Stephanie Baier:** Daily Affirmations for New Moms, Watch Me Grow: Baby Log Book, My Prayer Journal, Connected. Find on Amazon:

About the Author

Stephanie Baier is a mom, author, and holistic health enthusiast. She has two little girls, a stepdaughter and a biological daughter, and absolutely loves being their mom. After the birth of her baby, she struggled to find the time and energy to care for her health. Stephanie aims to share her experiences with new moms to help them know they are not alone on their journeys. With her background in Dietetics, she loves explaining nutrition concepts simply so that anyone can put 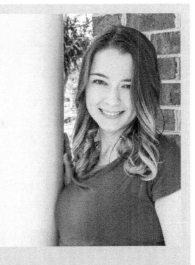 them into practice. She believes that a mother's health is affected by much more than her physical condition. Her mental health, relationship health, and self-care practices all tie into her overall well-being.

Made in United States
North Haven, CT
29 January 2024

48053214R10078